THE HIGH-PROTEIN
VEGAN COOKBOOK
FOR ATHLETES

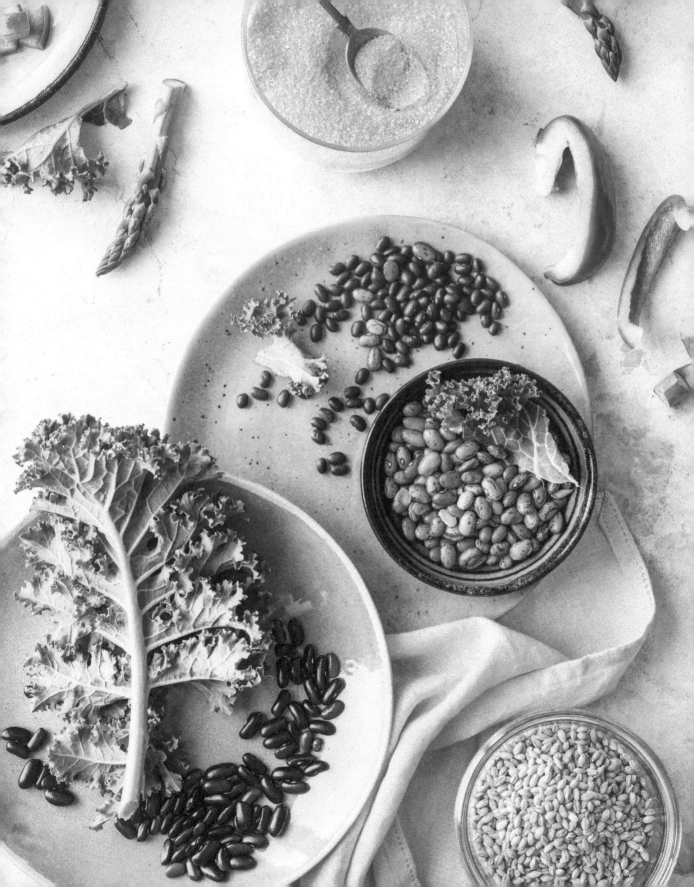

THE HIGH-PROTEIN VEGAN COOKBOOK FOR ATHLETES

70 Whole-Foods Recipes to Fuel Your Body

JENNA BRADDOCK, RD
IVY STARK

ROCKRIDGE
PRESS

For general information on our other products and services or to obtain technical support, please contact our Customer Care Department within the United States at (866) 744-2665, or outside the United States at (510) 253-0500.

Rockridge Press publishes its books in a variety of electronic and print formats. Some content that appears in print may not be available in electronic books, and vice versa.

TRADEMARKS: Rockridge Press and the Rockridge Press logo are trademarks or registered trademarks of Callisto Media Inc. and/or its affiliates, in the United States and other countries, and may not be used without written permission. All other trademarks are the property of their respective owners. Rockridge Press is not associated with any product or vendor mentioned in this book.

Interior and Cover Designer: Linda Snorina
Art Producer: Meg Baggott
Editor: Anna Pulley

Cover photo ©2021 Annie Martin

Nadine Greeff, ii; Annie Martin, vi; viii; Martí Sans/Stocksy Utd, x; Hélène Dujardin, 16; Darina Kopcok/Stocksy Utd, 34; News Life Media/StockFood USA, 52; Bauer Syndication/StockFood USA, 68; Denise Renée Schuster/StockFood USA, 90; Jan-Peter Westermann/StockFood USA, 116

Author photo courtesy of Michelle VanTine Photography

Cover image: Black Bean and Quinoa Meatballs with Marinara Sauce, page 102

Paperback ISBN: 978-1-64876-668-8
eBook ISBN: 978-1-64876-167-6

R0

FROM JENNA: *To the many athletes I've had the honor of working with over my career: your pursuit of excellence challenges me to do the same.*

FROM IVY: *To Charlie Brown, who never stopped trying to kick that football.*

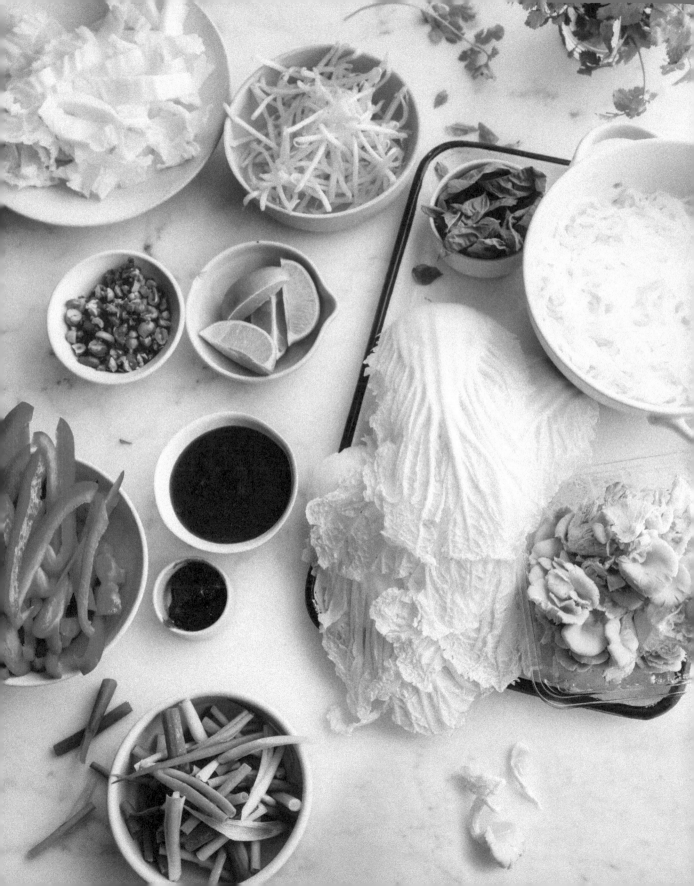

CONTENTS

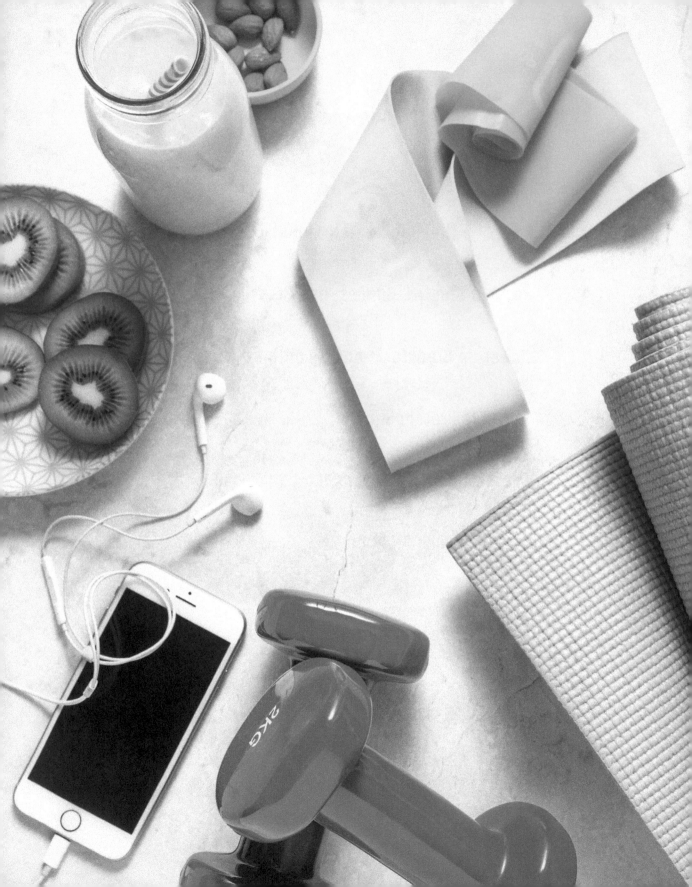

INTRODUCTION

If you're reading this book, it's safe to assume you're an athlete or physically active and interested in eating more plant-based foods. Welcome! I'm glad you chose this cookbook to help you on your path to better performance.

I'm a registered dietitian and Certified Specialist in Sports Dietetics (CSSD). From day one of my career, I've wanted to help athletes perform to the best of their ability. The human body is incredible, and fueling it well enables you to do more with it for longer.

I love working with athletes because they want to be their best and do what it takes to achieve their goals. Although this is a wonderful quality, it can work against them when it comes to trendy diets and supplements that promise game-changing results.

In recent years, plant-based eating has gained significant ground on the sports scene. Many high-level vegan athletes have emerged, such as Venus Williams, Alex Morgan, and Kyrie Irving, dispelling the myth that animal-based foods are a must for success. And even though some supplements and powders can help vegan athletes get the protein they need, you're here because eating a whole-foods, plant-based (WFPB) diet is important to you—and you want to learn how to do that better.

Following a high-protein, plant-based diet as an athlete is an excellent choice, but that doesn't mean it feels easy. Making the adjustment can be overwhelming. Given that, I encourage you to think of eating for performance as an experiment. Everything is trial and error with a spirit of curiosity. The goal is to land on a sweet spot of doable whole foods that taste great, feel good, and help you meet your performance goals.

In this book, you'll find a wealth of helpful information to equip you on your plant-based journey and make things a little easier. First, we'll dive into the basics of sports nutrition and fueling your body with plants. Then, you'll find 70 delicious, high-protein, plant-based recipes to help you eat well and prep your body for success.

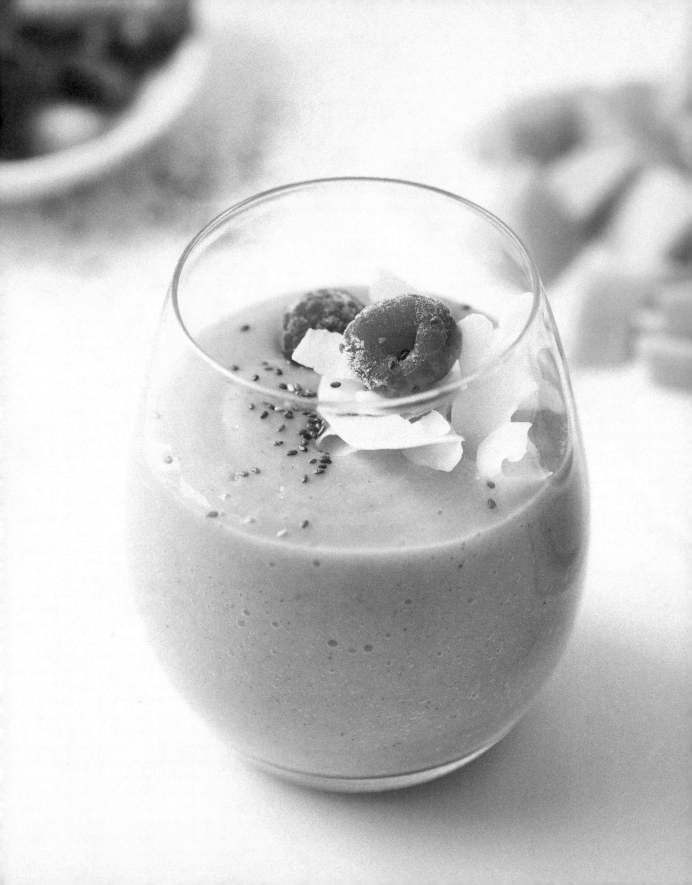

POWER UP
THE HIGH-PROTEIN,
PLANT-BASED WAY

"Should I go vegan?" is a question many athletes have asked me in the past couple of years. Maybe you're wondering this, too, or perhaps you've made the switch already to plant-based eating. Or maybe you're an athlete who wants to add more plant-based options to their overall diet. This book will help you regardless of where you're starting.

Nutrition is highly individualized—especially for athletes—but eating a predominantly plant-based diet is a positive change for just about everyone. It's possible to meet all the requirements of your body with a plant-based diet. Let's begin by looking at what your body needs to perform as a plant-based athlete.

Mango-Chia Recovery Shake
page 66

Yes, You Can Get All the Protein You Need from Plants

Plant-based eating will cover your carbohydrate bases—giving you the essential macronutrient for energy in an athlete's diet—because most plant foods contain at least some carbs. Protein, however, is the macronutrient often thought to be most "at risk." Decades ago, this may have been true, but with new research and greater availability of plant-based foods, it's possible to get the protein you need while eating a vegan diet.

You're likely coming to this book with some foundational knowledge of sports nutrition and plant-based eating, so we're not going to start from scratch. This book is intended to be a creative addition to your high-protein eating plan, not the starting place for building your performance diet. However, your questions about protein needs, vegan protein sources, and delicious ways to achieve high-protein meals and snacks will be answered. If you want more information on general sports nutrition, visit the Resources section at the end of this book (see page 127).

What Do We Mean by High-Protein?

The amount of protein you need as an athlete is a highly debated topic in scientific research. The most recent Dietary Guidelines for Americans recommend adults 19 and up get 10 to 30 percent of their total calories from protein, or about 0.8g/kg of body weight, but athletes usually need more protein than that, specifically for building and maintaining lean muscle. Being a vegan athlete adds another layer to protein needs, since plant-based proteins can be less bioavailable (readily absorbed by the body) than animal sources. That said, recent research published in *Nutrients* found a higher intake of plant-based protein may attenuate this problem.

Many studies have looked at exactly how many grams of protein per meal are ideal for stimulating and maintaining muscle growth. Ultimately, protein needs are highly individualized, based on your genetics, goals, and sport. Studies show that many people, not just athletes, can benefit from meals containing anywhere from 20 to 60 grams of protein.

For the purposes of this book, "high-protein" refers to vegan meals created with protein-rich ingredients that contain 20 to 30 grams of protein per serving. I want to equip you with a variety of recipes to help meet the demands of your training. Research suggests that spreading protein intake evenly throughout the day is ideal for meeting athletes' needs.

In the past, vegetarian and vegan athletes were advised to complement their plant-based protein choices to get all the essential amino acids. Current information recommends focusing on eating a wide variety of plant foods, which will more than likely provide what you need.

THE LOWDOWN ON PROTEIN POWDERS

Many athletes, both vegan and not, believe they must supplement their diets with protein powder. This isn't necessarily true, since it's possible to meet your needs as an athlete through food, and you should try to do so. However, the benefit of protein powders is significant when you consider the barriers most athletes face when fueling only through foods. Time, budget, schedule, access, convenience, and very high protein needs are reasons why you might consider including a protein supplement in your routine.

There are a lot of options for vegan protein powders, and it's easy to be misled. Soy and pea proteins are my favorite single-source options for vegan athletes, since they have good amino acid profiles and research studies show they positively impact muscle. Pea is a perfect option for athletes who are allergic to soy, and you'll find a recipe for Pea Protein Powder on page 18. In terms of store-bought options, look for a soy or pea protein isolate with a minimal ingredient list. Another strategy is to look for a vegan protein that is a blend of many sources (like pea, soy, and rice) to help get a variety of essential amino acids.

Nutrition for Athletes 101

Before taking a deep dive into all protein does for athletes, here's a quick refresher on basic sports nutrition.

Macronutrients

Macronutrients, or macros, are the nutrients that provide the energy that fuels the body. There are three main macro categories: carbohydrates, protein, and fat. Although it's easy to think of foods as being from only one macro category, it's important to remember that many foods are a blend of energy sources.

Carbohydrates are a readily available fuel source for the body. They are crucial for athletes, since carb quantity and timing play critical roles in improving performance. Vegan athletes may have a naturally higher intake of carbohydrates, which is perfectly acceptable.

Carbohydrates are found in many foods, including fruits, vegetables, grains and flours, sugars and sweeteners, legumes, nuts, seeds, and dairy alternatives.

Protein plays a minor role in supplying energy to an active body. It's vital for providing the nutrients needed to maintain, repair, and build muscle tissue. When protein is digested, it's broken down into the smaller amino acids used to build tissue—including muscle—throughout the body. Amino acids are not stored idly in the body, waiting to be utilized in times of need, so it is necessary to eat protein regularly. Eating enough protein is a concern for athletes because their needs are elevated based on the demands of their training and their goals for their bodies.

Whereas carbohydrates and protein have clear roles in providing energy or physiological functioning, fat dips its toes into both categories. **Fat** is a significant energy source and plays a role in a wide array of functions within the body. Athletes can rely on fat to help them meet high energy needs, deliver satiety after eating, and make food taste better. An adequate amount of essential fats (like omega-3s) can promote optimal functioning of the vascular, endocrine, inflammatory, and central nervous systems. It's important to ensure regular intake of plant-based fats like nuts, olives, avocados, seeds, and certain oils. Omega-3 fats can be found in plant foods like flax, hemp, pumpkin seeds, and sea algae.

Each athlete should consider their unique macronutrient needs based on their body, sport, goals, training, competition schedule, and health history. The ideal way to determine your unique needs is to work with a registered dietitian who is also a certified specialist in sports dietetics (CSSD). You can find one by using the Academy of Nutrition and Dietetics's Find a Nutrition Expert tool. You can also take a do-it-yourself approach using free online tools like MyFitnessPal.com, but these are not necessarily designed with athletes in mind.

Key Micronutrients

Vitamins and minerals are micronutrients—compounds required in smaller amounts that do not provide energy to the body. Micronutrients are involved in everything from growth and development to energy metabolism and muscle function.

Almost all whole foods contain micronutrients, so eating a diverse diet is ideal. It's debatable whether athletes have a greater need for micronutrients. Since animal protein contains high levels of some important vitamins and minerals, plant-based athletes need a plan to meet their needs.

Here is a list of important micronutrients for plant-based athletes:

IRON is essential for moving oxygen through the body to working muscles. Low iron levels, common in female athletes, can cause unexplained fatigue and poor performance. The most bioavailable form of iron is found in animal proteins, so be conscientious about iron intake. Eat high-iron foods with a source of vitamin C to boost absorption.
Sources: spinach, asparagus, Swiss chard, lentils, sesame seeds, tofu, raisins, whole grains

ZINC plays a role in hundreds of metabolic processes and is necessary for a strong immune system. Plant-based sources of zinc are not as bioavailable as animal sources, plus phytates in plants can make absorption of zinc even harder. Zinc bioavailability can be enhanced by soaking or sprouting grains (page 31), seeds, and beans to reduce phytates.
Sources: beans, nuts, seeds, whole grains, fortified cereals, soy products

OMEGA-3 FATTY ACIDS include DHA, EPA, and ALA and are important for maintaining heart and brain health and attenuating exercise-related inflammation.
Sources: algae, flaxseed, hemp seeds, walnuts

VITAMIN D is essential for bone health, immune function, regulation of inflammation, and muscle function. Low vitamin D blood levels are common, so get your levels checked, and discuss with a healthcare provider whether supplementation is necessary.
Sources: fortified vegan spreads, breakfast cereals, fortified plant-based milk and juices, sun-dried mushrooms

CALCIUM is crucial for ensuring bone and muscle health. Luckily, plant-based calcium sources can easily meet an athlete's needs.
Sources: tofu processed with calcium, dark leafy greens (like bok choy and kale), nuts, seeds, kidney beans, fortified plant-based milk

VITAMIN C aids in the absorption of both iron and zinc and supports immune function.
Sources: Brussels sprouts, broccoli, peppers, oranges, papaya, guava

VITAMIN B$_{12}$ is a nutrient that vegans need to watch because the active form is found almost exclusively in animal foods. A deficiency of B$_{12}$ can cause fatigue and irregular heartbeat. A supplement can be a helpful option.
Sources: nutritional yeast, fortified breakfast cereals, fortified plant-based milk, yogurt

How Protein Enhances Your Athletic Performance

It's common knowledge, especially among athletes, that protein helps build muscle. Beyond that, there's often not a deep understanding of exactly why protein is important for athletic performance. Let's learn more about protein and look at a cheat sheet for determining your needs.

Protein for Energy and Endurance

Protein can be used as a fuel source during activity, especially during endurance exercise. This is not necessarily a "good" or "bad" thing, but it can be negative if muscle tissue is broken down to provide energy too much or too often. Eating adequate protein ensures that your body has ample amino acids to rebuild any lost tissue, which ultimately helps you remain healthy and strong.

AWESOME AMINO ACIDS

Amino acids are the building blocks of all the protein structures found in the human body and are classified as essential or non-essential. Nonessential amino acids are made within the human body by its own mechanics. The body cannot produce the nine essential amino acids, so they need to be consumed through food sources. Here are the main ones to pay attention to:

Branch chain amino acids leucine, isoleucine, and valine all play critical roles in metabolic function, muscle building, and recovery.
Sources: wheat protein, oats, soybeans, lentils, seeds

Lysine is essential for growth and tissue repair. It promotes calcium uptake, improves the immune system, and is essential for collagen formation.
Sources: beans, legumes, soy products such as tofu and soy milk

Methionine is required for tissue repair and growth and plays a pivotal role in improving and strengthening hair, skin, and nails. It also protects our cells from pollutants, slows the aging of cells, and is involved in multiple detoxifying processes.
Sources: Brazil nuts, sesame seeds, oats

Threonine has been shown to decrease symptoms of depression and anxiety and prevent fat buildup in the liver. It's also involved in forming many proteins, such as collagen, tooth enamel, and elastin.
Sources: white beans and soy products, including tofu and edamame

To ensure that protein is used for building the body and not for regularly providing energy, it's essential for athletes to eat the correct quantity of food to match their training demands. This concept is called energy availability and is an important starting point for athletes to ensure that their bodies are properly fueled. So, carefully consider the foods you eat or do not eat, evaluating whether each provides value or not to *your* body and training.

Protein needs are not as commonly discussed with endurance athletes because of the emphasis on leanness, adequate calories, and carbohydrate intake. Although endurance athletes may not consider protein for rebuilding muscle tissue, they need protein to repair the tissue broken down through prolonged exercise and training.

Protein for Strength and Muscle Building

Protein is most associated with its ability to help your body build muscle. When you eat a protein containing all the amino acids, your body has the building blocks to fully respond to training. A large body of evidence shows that eating protein can help stimulate muscle growth and increase the rate at which that happens post-workout. Whether your goal is to build new muscle or maintain what you already have, eating enough protein is imperative for optimal performance.

Protein for Lowering Body Fat

Historically, periods of lowering body weight, body fat, or both were thought to benefit certain athletes. However, I encourage all athletes and coaches to focus on performance and not just body composition. Being a certain weight or having a certain body fat percentage does not guarantee anything and can perpetuate unhealthy and even harmful practices among athletes.

With that said, if lowering body fat is a constructive change for you as an athlete, protein can play a powerful role in that process. According to a 2018 review paper by researchers at McMaster University, increasing protein intake to 1.6 to 2.4g/kg body weight per day is suggested during periods of fat loss to help maintain lean muscle tissue and provide satiety in meals.

Protein for Recovery

There's a vast body of research about the timing of eating protein and how it impacts muscle growth, performance, and recovery. Experimenting with protein timing before and after training could produce better outcomes and is a critical component of a tight nutrition plan. Ultimately, though, eating protein throughout the day, shortly after a workout, and before bed is key to gaining the full benefits of protein for recovery and muscle growth.

Protein for Immunity

A strong immune system is a vital component of sports performance. Intense training periods can compromise an athlete's immune system, increasing their susceptibility to illness. Adequate intake of certain amino acids can help increase immune system activity and may help fight infection. This means fewer missed days and an overall stronger body.

Protein Needs Cheat Sheet

The protein needs of athletes are highly individualized and can vary greatly based on training schedule, competition, age, rest days, and personal goals. These recommendations are a guide for experimenting with your personal needs.

ATHLETIC NEED	RECOMMENDED PROTEIN INTAKE (G/KG)
Endurance Training	1.2–1.6g/kg/day
Strength Training	1.6–2.0g/kg/day
Muscle Building/Bodybuilding	1.6–2.2g/kg/day
Rest/Recovery Days	1.0–2.0g/kg/day

The Wide World of Plant-Based Protein

A powerful strategy for a plant-powered athlete is to eat a wide variety of foods. This helps ensure that your intake of the essential amino acids and other nutrients is adequate to promote health and performance. No matter where you are on the spectrum of plant-based eating, including a wide variety of foods keeps meals exciting and balanced.

There are well-known plant-based protein sources, like soy, but there are also some "sneakier" or unexpected sources. Although it is not meant to be comprehensive, the following chart includes examples of high-protein plant foods that might not be on your radar.

PLANT-BASED PROTEIN SOURCES

FOOD	SERVING	PROTEIN	FAT	CARBS
QUINOA (DRY)	½ cup	12g	5g	55g
TOFU	100g	8.1g	4.7g	1.7g
CHICKPEAS	1 cup	15g	4.2g	45g
EDAMAME	½ cup	9.2g	4g	7g
PEANUT BUTTER	2 tablespoons	7g	16g	7.7g
HEMP SEEDS	2 tablespoons	6.3g	10g	1.7g
LENTILS (COOKED)	½ cup	9g	0.4g	20g
HULLED BARLEY	1 cup	5.7g	1g	33g
TAHINI	1 tablespoon	2.6g	8g	3.2g
NUTRITIONAL YEAST	2 tablespoons	7.6g	1.2g	6.3g
PEAS	½ cup	4.3g	0.15g	12g
BROWN RICE	1 cup	5g	1.6g	46g
ROLLED OATS (DRY)	½ cup	5.3g	2.6g	27g
WHOLE-WHEAT BREAD	2 slices	8g	2.2g	28g
BLACK BEANS (COOKED)	½ cup	8g	0.5g	23g
SOY MILK	1 cup	7g	4g	8g
CHIA SEEDS	2 tablespoons	4g	7.4g	10g

Source: nutritionix.com

SORTING THROUGH
THE SOY CONTROVERSY

Soy protein, found in edamame, tofu, miso, tempeh, and soy milk, is considered a primary protein source for many vegans. However, there's controversy around the effectiveness and safety of soy protein for athletes.

A meta-analysis published in the *International Journal of Sport Nutrition and Exercise Metabolism* concluded that although whey protein has a greater effect on muscle synthesis, soy protein has similar effects on lean body mass and strength during resistance exercise training. This is likely due to the branched-chain amino acid leucine, found in higher amounts in whey protein. Though other forms of protein may result in greater muscle growth, soy protein, compared to a placebo, has been found to effectively enhance muscle recovery and reduce muscle damage.

Soy protein contains a phytoestrogen called isoflavone, which is why the effects of soy on hormones and hormone signaling mechanisms are questioned. Some studies have shown that increased consumption of soy protein may lead to earlier onset of puberty in boys, and others have shown no change in sexual maturation in boys and girls. In adults, soy protein has been shown to have no effect on estrogen, specifically estradiol, or free testosterone, but may reduce circulating testosterone in a small percentage of people.

Overall, soy protein is one of the few plant-based complete proteins containing all essential amino acids. There is limited current evidence to support negative effects of soy on athletic performance. Soy protein should be included in a balanced vegan diet.

Stocking Your High-Protein Plant-Based Kitchen

A well-stocked kitchen makes your life as a busy athlete easier and more manageable. This section outlines the essential foods and equipment to make the recipes in this book.

Power Proteins

EDAMAME: Frozen, fresh, or roasted edamame are a quick, easy protein addition to any meal. Buy them frozen in the pod or shelled.

FLAVORED PROTEIN POWDERS: This cookbook includes recipes to make protein powder, but buying this ingredient is also acceptable. Different flavors, such as chocolate, can be kept on hand for easy prep.

HIGH-PROTEIN PASTA: Pasta is an awesome base for meals. There are many types, including products made with high-protein bean flours.

LENTILS: Lentils are a superpowered protein option and very versatile. Buy them dried, precooked in a pouch, or canned.

NUTS AND NUT BUTTERS: Enjoy a wide variety of nuts to provide different amino acids, nutrients, and healthy fats. Look for nuts and nut butters in bulk to save money.

PUMPKIN SEEDS: Pumpkin seeds offer protein, essential nutrients, and amino acids. Buy them in bulk at wholesale stores. They may also be called pepitas.

SOY MILK PRODUCTS: Look for soy milk–based products like yogurt and creamer. Store-bought soy milk is budget friendly and is available in shelf-stable cartons.

WHOLE GRAINS: Enjoy a wide variety of whole grains, including oats, farro, barley, wild rice, and more. Look for frozen and quick-cooking options to make meals faster.

Other Staples

100% FRUIT JUICE: This staple can be an easy source of nutrients and energy for athletes who need it. Each kind has unique benefits, like tart cherry juice for muscle soreness and sleep or orange juice for added calcium or vitamin D.

BERRIES: Fresh, canned in juice, or frozen berries can aid in recovery and immune function.

GREEN VEGETABLES: Try spinach, kale, chard, broccoli, green peppers, Brussels sprouts, cabbage, cucumbers, and zucchini. Fresh, frozen, and canned are all excellent options.

HERBS AND SPICES: Herbs and spices add excitement to meals. Try basil, oregano, thyme, chili powder, paprika, cumin, and others.

Equipment and Tools

BAKING SHEETS: Quality rimmed baking sheets (quarter, half, and full) are essential for jobs big and small.

BOWLS: Look for a minimum of three nested bowls in a material that suits your lifestyle.

BOX GRATER: I recommend box graters with a big handle for holding and a measuring cup attachment.

CASSEROLE DISHES: 8-inch square and 9-by-13-inch are perfect for many recipes in this book.

DUTCH OVEN: This pot can do it all, from stovetop to oven.

FINE-MESH SIEVE (OR CHEESECLOTH): You'll need this to drain off excess liquid, a technique often used in this book.

HIGH-SPEED BLENDER OR FOOD PROCESSOR: A strong, durable blender with a wide range of programs is essential. A food processor can be faster and more appropriate for some recipes (like Vegan Soft Cheese, page 24).

JARS WITH LIDS: A set of wide-mouth glass jars (12- to 16-ounce) for oats, puddings, smoothies, and more will come in handy.

MUFFIN TIN: Choose a lighter-colored metal for more even cooking.

SKILLET: Look for large and small ones made of durable material such as stainless steel or cast iron.

How to Use This Book to Fit Your Lifestyle

The recipes in this book are designed to be high in plant-based protein or to serve as bases for building high-protein meals and snacks. You'll see familiar ingredients used in new and unique ways, so you won't get bored. There is also guidance on when certain recipes may be beneficial to your training. Look for labels at the top of each recipe to show which recipes will work best for you.

The Skinny on the Recipes

If your plate is already full of responsibilities, then you've come to the right place. This book contains recipes that are easy to execute, and most have 12 ingredients or fewer. Some recipes are more time-consuming, but the work is well worth it. The more you practice, the quicker you'll whip them up!

Each recipe contains at least one tip, including cooking advice, storage instructions for leftovers, or the option to swap something out based on preference. Nutrition facts are also included to guide athletes who find this information helpful for tracking macros or micros.

Read the Labels

The recipes include four athletic performance labels: **HIGH-CARB, LOW-CARB, RECOVERY BOOST,** and **QUENCH THE HUNGER.** High-Carb recipes are for when you need more energy. Low-Carb are naturally lower in carbs. Recovery Boost are particularly beneficial for recovery after tough workouts. And Quench the Hunger are filling meals that are well rounded in macronutrients. Also, we've included gluten-free and nut-free labels for people who have additional dietary concerns. Always check ingredient packaging for gluten-free labeling in order to ensure that foods, especially oats, were processed in a completely gluten-free facility.

The Double Up and Store It Method

If you are like many of the athletes I've worked with, the intention to eat well is there, but time is not always in your favor. We've got your back here. Many recipes can be stored for future meals and doubled to save time and energy. Look for storage and reheating info tips to guide you on the best way to keep your hard work and delicious meals fresh.

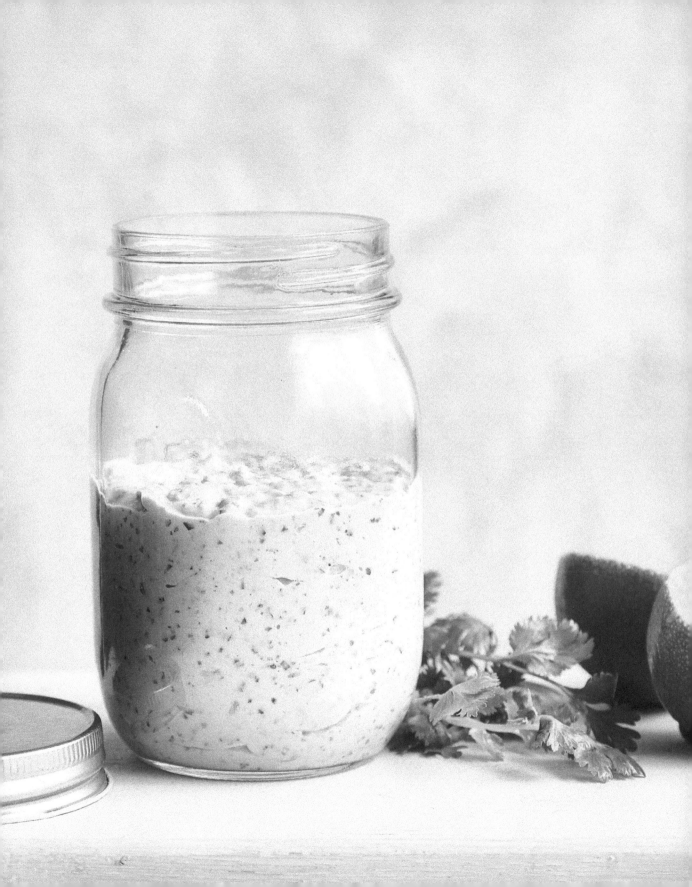

PROTEIN STAPLES, SAUCES, AND DRESSINGS

This chapter is like your basic training course to set up a healthy and strong vegan diet. Many staples like protein powder and tofu are available in most grocery stores, but making them yourself is easy and, in the end, saves time and money. Stocking whole-food staples in the kitchen allows you to quickly put together healthy vegan meals without using processed foods. Most of these recipes require little active time and inexpensive ingredients. As you become more familiar with the recipes, use them to batch-cook and meal prep. You'll then be fully equipped to handle the ebbs and flows of your training schedule and life in general.

Green Goddess Dressing
page 28

PEA PROTEIN POWDER

GLUTEN-FREE

NUT-FREE

RECOVERY BOOST

MAKES 1 CUP

PREP TIME: 10 minutes

1 cup dried split peas

This allergen-friendly and easy-to-digest protein powder comes together in minutes. Pea protein powder is naturally vegan, budget friendly, and a great way to add a protein kick to your smoothies, baked goods, soups, and sauces.

1. Put the peas in a dry blender or food processor and cover tightly with the lid. Process until the peas are reduced to a fine powder. Wait a moment before removing the lid to allow the powder to settle, so you won't have a powder cloud mess.

2. Using a fine-mesh strainer, sift the processed peas into a bowl, placing any large pieces that remain in the strainer back in the blender for another 3 minutes and sifting again until you have a fine powder.

   STORAGE: Refrigerate in an airtight container for up to 1 week, or freeze for up to 6 months.

   VARIATION: For extra flavor, add a spoonful of cocoa, vanilla bean, or maca powder. Cinnamon and a touch of coconut sugar also make great add-ins for a bit of sweetness.

   PER SERVING (2 TABLESPOONS): Calories: 87; Protein: 8g; Total fat: 0g; Carbohydrates: 16g; Fiber: 6g; Calcium: 9mg; Vitamin D: 0mg; Vitamin B_{12}: 0mg; Iron: 1mg; Zinc: 1mg

   MACROS: Protein 23%; Carbs 74%; Fat 3%

5-SEED PROTEIN POWDER

GLUTEN-FREE
NUT-FREE
QUENCH THE HUNGER
RECOVERY BOOST

MAKES 2 CUPS

PREP TIME: 15 minutes

2 tablespoons chia seeds

3 tablespoons hemp seeds

¼ cup brown rice powder

¼ cup pumpkin seeds

¼ cup ground flaxseed

⅓ cup **Pea Protein Powder (page 18) or store-bought protein powder**

This recipe comes from a time-saving experiment when making breakfast smoothies. Along with protein powder, I added seeds and brown rice powder to smoothies for extra protein. I ended up with multiple jars of ingredients, extra time spent measuring, and a mess. I decided to grind everything ahead of time and create this all-in-one powder.

1. In a dry high-speed blender or food processor, separately process the chia seeds, hemp seeds, brown rice powder, pumpkin seeds, and flaxseed until they turn to a fine powder.

2. Sift each through a fine-mesh strainer into a bowl.

3. Add the protein powder, stirring to thoroughly combine.

STORAGE: Refrigerate in an airtight container for up to 1 week, or freeze for up to 6 months.

SERVING TIP: Protein powder is not just for smoothies; this flavorful 5-seed blend can be tossed into a vegetable stir-fry, sprinkled over a grain bowl, or stirred into a soup for extra protein.

PER SERVING (¼ CUP): Calories: 132; Protein: 6g; Total fat: 6g; Carbohydrates: 12g; Fiber: 4g; Calcium: 41mg; Vitamin D: 0mg; Vitamin B_{12}: 0mg; Iron: 2mg; Zinc: 0mg

MACROS: Protein 15%; Carbs 30%; Fat 55%

BASIC SEITAN

LOW-CARB

NUT-FREE

QUENCH THE HUNGER

SERVES 2

PREP TIME: 15 minutes
COOK TIME: 1 hour
15 minutes, plus overnight to set

1 tablespoon olive oil
1 large yellow or white onion, diced
⅓ teaspoon sea salt
2 garlic cloves, minced
1 teaspoon paprika
½ teaspoon everything seasoning blend like (Trader Joe's 21 Seasoning Salute) or Old Bay
1 cup low-sodium vegetable stock
¼ cup chickpea flour
2 tablespoons nutritional yeast
2 tablespoons tomato paste
1 tablespoon soy sauce (optional; omit for soy-free)
1½ cups vital wheat gluten

Seitan is one of the most versatile and "meatiest" meat substitutes. This ingredient can be sliced, grilled, ground, and used in chili, stews, or stir-fries. The process to make seitan is a little involved, but the homemade results are well worth it.

1. In a large skillet, heat the oil over medium heat.

2. Add the onion and salt. Sauté for 4 to 6 minutes, until the onion has softened slightly and becomes translucent.

3. Reduce the heat to medium-low. Add the garlic and stir. Cook for about 2 minutes, until the garlic is softened and fragrant, but do not let it brown.

4. Add the paprika and seasoning blend. Stir and cook for 1 minute or until the aromas are released. Remove from the heat.

5. Using a large spoon, transfer the onion-garlic mixture to a food processor.

6. Add the stock, chickpea flour, nutritional yeast, tomato paste, and soy sauce (if using). Blend until smooth. Transfer to a large bowl.

7. Fold in the wheat gluten, then stir until incorporated. Once it is combined, knead the mixture for about 2 minutes or until firm and bouncy.

8. Prepare the steamer. (See the tip for a simple steamer setup.) Form the dough into a loaf shape and roll it up tightly in a piece of aluminum foil, twisting the ends tightly to secure. Depending on the size of your steamer, prepare 2 loaves if needed.

9. Once the water is boiling, put the dough in the steamer and steam for 1 hour, carefully turning it over with a spoon or tongs after 30 minutes. Remove from the heat. Let cool to room temperature, then unwrap and refrigerate in an airtight container or bag for at least 8 hours to overnight. To keep the seitan from drying out, slice as needed for recipes.

STORAGE: Refrigerate the seitan in log form for 1 week, or freeze for 1 month.

COOKING TIP: To make a steamer, place a small mesh colander in a saucepan with a lid over 1 inch of boiling water.

PER SERVING: Calories: 396; Protein: 86g; Total fat: 10g; Carbohydrates: 34g; Fiber: 4g; Calcium: 192mg; Vitamin D: 0mg; Vitamin B$_{12}$: 0mg; Iron: 7mg; Zinc: 2mg

MACROS: Protein 62%; Carbs 23%; Fat 15%

FRESH TOFU AND SOY MILK

GLUTEN-FREE

NUT-FREE

RECOVERY BOOST

SERVES 2

PREP TIME: 15 minutes, plus overnight to soak

COOK TIME: 1 hour

8 ounces dried soybeans

9½ cups water, plus more for soaking the beans, divided

1½ teaspoons nigari flakes

> **STORAGE:** If you're going to store the tofu for more than 1 day, put some cool water in its storage container and refrigerate. The soy milk keeps for up to 5 days in the refrigerator.

> **PREP TIP:** If you plan to prepare tofu often, a tofu mold is a good and inexpensive purchase. Or create a simple mold with a 1-quart strawberry container. I use a small colander with a plate to cover, which makes dome-shaped tofu.

Make tofu at home? Yes, you can! Nigari flakes are the coagulant used to turn soy milk into tofu, and they can be purchased at health food stores or online. If you're just making fresh soy milk, follow the recipe to step 5, and enjoy!

1. To make the soy milk, put the soybeans in a large bowl and cover with 2 inches of cold water. Cover with plastic wrap and let sit at room temperature overnight. After soaking, the soybeans should plump up considerably. Drain and rinse with cold water.

2. Transfer 1 cup of the soybeans to a blender. Add 3 cups of water. Blend on high speed for about 1 minute, until the mixture is smooth and milky white. Pour the soy milk into a large, deep stockpot. Repeat with the remaining soybeans.

3. Bring the soy milk to a simmer over medium heat, stirring frequently. Reduce the heat to medium-low. Continue to simmer for 10 minutes. Remove from the heat.

4. Place a fine-mesh strainer over a large bowl or pot. Line the strainer with a clean kitchen towel or a triple layer of cheesecloth.

5. Ladle the soy milk into the strainer, letting the milk drain into the bowl. Bring the edges of the towel together to form a sack and twist to squeeze out as much of the milk as possible. Discard the remaining pulp.

6. To make the tofu: pour the soy milk back into the stockpot. Bring to a boil over medium-high heat. Remove from the heat. Let sit for 3 to 4 minutes, stirring occasionally to prevent a skin from forming.

7. Meanwhile, in a small bowl, dissolve the nigari in ½ cup of water.

8. While stirring, pour about one-third of the nigari mixture into the soy milk. Continue to stir for about 15 seconds. Pour another third of the nigari into the soy milk. Cover and let rest for 3 minutes. Uncover the pot. The milk should be curdling.

9. Sprinkle the remaining nigari over the top, and gently stir it into the milk, trying not to disturb the curds. Cover and let rest for 3 minutes.

10. Uncover the pot. If the curds have separated from the clear yellow liquid whey, you're ready for the next step. If you see still see milky areas in the pot, gently give them a stir, cover, and let sit for another 3 minutes.

11. While the soy milk is curdling, set up the tofu mold (see tip for details) on a rimmed baking sheet. Line the mold with fine cheesecloth.

12. Using a spoon, pour a bit of whey into the mold to moisten the cloth.

13. Using a slotted spoon, gently transfer the curds to the mold, trying to keep the curds as intact as possible. Once all the curds have been transferred, fold the cloth over them. Place the lid or a plate on top of the cloth, then place a weight on the lid. A can of tomatoes will work well as a weight.

14. Let the tofu rest under the weight until it has reached the texture you desire. For medium tofu, about 15 minutes or until it's about half its original height. For firm tofu, 30 to 45 minutes and about one-third of its original height. Once the firmness is correct, remove the weight, lid, and mold. Let the tofu rest, wrapped in the cloth, until it has reached room temperature.

15. Unwrap the tofu and refrigerate until you're ready to eat.

PER SERVING (1 CUP): Calories: 60; Protein: 7g; Total fat: 3g; Carbohydrates: 3g; Fiber: 1g; Calcium: 299mg; Vitamin D: 0mg; Vitamin B$_{12}$: 3mg; Iron: 1mg; Zinc: 1mg

MACROS: Protein 35%; Carbs 20%; Fat 45%

VEGAN SOFT CHEESE

MAKES 1 POUND

PREP TIME: 5 minutes, plus 8 hours to soak and 1 to 2 days to ferment

2 cups organic
  raw cashews
½ cup water
2 tablespoons
  vegan yogurt
¼ teaspoon sea salt

It's simple to make vegan cheese at home with a few ingredients. This basic recipe can be used as a spread for toast or in recipes like lasagna. You'll see it in many other recipes in this book. You can also dress your cheese up with herbs, spices, nuts, roasted garlic, or sun-dried tomatoes for a protein-packed snack with crackers or raw veggies.

1. Put the cashews in a medium bowl and cover with 2 inches of water. Cover with plastic wrap and soak at room temperature for at least 8 hours to overnight. Drain.

2. Put the cashews, water, yogurt, and salt in a food processor. Process until smooth and creamy. Transfer to a glass bowl. Cover tightly and let rest at room temperature for 24 to 48 hours to ferment. Serve or refrigerate.

STORAGE: This keeps in a sealed container for 2 weeks in the refrigerator or 4 months in the freezer.

SERVING TIP: This vegan soft cheese can be used anywhere you would use cream cheese or ricotta cheese.

PER SERVING (2 OUNCES): Calories: 211; Protein: 7g; Total fat: 17g; Carbohydrates: 12g; Fiber: 1g; Calcium: 19mg; Vitamin D: 0mg; Vitamin B_{12}: 0mg; Iron: 3mg; Zinc: 2mg

MACROS: Protein 11%; Carbs 24%; Fat 65%

VEGAN MAYONNAISE

GLUTEN-FREE

LOW-CARB

NUT-FREE

QUENCH THE HUNGER

MAKES 1 CUP

PREP TIME: 5 minutes

½ cup avocado oil or any
  neutral-flavored oil

¼ cup soy milk

1 teaspoon apple
  cider vinegar

1 teaspoon freshly
  squeezed lemon juice

1 teaspoon Dijon mustard

½ teaspoon sea salt, plus
  more as needed

⅛ teaspoon ground
  turmeric

Technically, this isn't a mayonnaise because it doesn't contain egg, but this tangy, creamy, and rich spread is perfect for sandwiches or salads or as a base for dressings or sauces. It can be flavored any way you'd like; I like to add chipotle in adobo and tarragon. This recipe can be made in a snap and used anywhere you would use regular mayonnaise.

Put the oil, soy milk, vinegar, lemon juice, mustard, salt, and turmeric in a high-speed blender or food processor. Process at high speed for about 2 minutes, until the mixture emulsifies and is thick and creamy. Adjust the seasoning with salt as desired.

STORAGE: Refrigerate in an airtight container for 7 to 10 days.

VARIATION: Add more acidity with additional apple cider vinegar or lemon juice and sea salt. Blend in your favorite herb or combination of herbs for a delicious herb mayonnaise.

PER SERVING (1 TABLESPOON): Calories: 62; Protein: 0g; Total fat: 7g; Carbohydrates: 0g; Fiber: 0g; Calcium: 5mg; Vitamin D: 0mg; Vitamin B_{12}: 0mg; Iron: 0mg; Zinc: 0mg

MACROS: Protein 1%; Carbs 1%; Fat 98%

ALMOND MILK YOGURT

MAKES 2 CUPS

PREP TIME: 15 minutes, plus 1 to 2 days to ferment

2 cups organic unsweet-
ened almond milk

Tiny pinch agar powder

2 vegan-friendly probi-
otic capsules (ensure
that they do not contain
prebiotic fiber), such
as Jarrow Probiotic
10 Billion

Almond milk yogurt is one of my favorite foods. It can be enjoyed on its own, whipped for a dessert topping, or drizzled on a baked sweet potato as a sour cream substitute. It's easy to make, and the taste of homemade is incomparable. Agar powder is a vegan gelatin substance that can be found at larger grocery stores, at health food stores, and online.

1. Put the almond milk and agar powder in a small saucepan. Stir to combine. Bring to a boil over medium heat.

2. Reduce the heat to low. Simmer for 5 minutes. Remove from the heat. Pour the almond milk into a sterilized dry glass jar or bowl. Let cool completely until the consistency resembles yogurt.

3. Empty the probiotic capsules into the yogurt and stir using a wooden spoon. (Do not use a metal spoon, since that can react negatively with the probiotics.) Stir until creamy, smooth, and thoroughly combined.

4. Cover the mixture with cheesecloth or a clean kitchen towel and secure using a rubber band or kitchen twine.

5. Let the yogurt activate for at least 24 hours and up to 48 hours in a warm place; the longer it rests, the tangier the yogurt will be. In warmer climates and summer, it's easy to make yogurt if your house is warm, but in cooler climates and winter, place the yogurt in the oven with the light on (no flame) to activate.

6. Once the yogurt has reached the desired tanginess and thickness, cover tightly with a lid or plastic wrap and refrigerate until cold.

STORAGE: Refrigerate in an airtight container for up to 1 week.

VARIATION: Enjoy this delicious yogurt plain, or add protein powder, fruit, nuts, shredded coconut, and a bit of sweetener like maple syrup or vanilla.

PER SERVING (½ CUP): Calories: 15; Protein: 0g; Total fat: 1g; Carbohydrates: 0g; Fiber: 0g; Calcium: 225mg; Vitamin D: 1mg; Vitamin B_{12}: 0mg; Iron: 0mg; Zinc: 0mg

MACROS: Protein 20%; Carbs 10%; Fat 70%

GREEN GODDESS DRESSING

GLUTEN-FREE

LOW-CARB

NUT-FREE

MAKES 1 QUART

PREP TIME: 10 minutes

1 ripe avocado, peeled, pitted, and diced

¾ cup silken tofu

3 tablespoons avocado oil

3 tablespoons freshly squeezed lime juice

Grated zest of 2 limes

1½ teaspoons Dijon mustard

1 large garlic clove

2 tarragon sprigs, chopped

2 parsley sprigs, chopped

2 basil sprigs, chopped

2 teaspoons freshly ground black pepper

1 teaspoon sea salt, plus more as needed

Green goddess dressing is the ultimate addition for a great salad. This recipe contains quite a few ingredients, but they are totally worth it to create a dressing that really wows your taste buds. Don't just limit this goodness to salad; use it as a dip, spread it on sandwiches, or even toss it in pasta dishes.

Put the avocado, tofu, oil, lime juice, lime zest, mustard, garlic, tarragon, parsley, basil, pepper, and salt in a blender or food processor. Puree until smooth. Adjust the seasoning with salt as needed. Use the dressing immediately, or put it in a covered container and refrigerate.

STORAGE: Refrigerate in an airtight container for up to 3 days.

SERVING TIP: Green goddess is great used as a cool sauce for grilled tofu or seitan, drizzled over grilled vegetables, or as a mix-in for hummus.

PER SERVING (2 TABLESPOONS): Calories: 27; Protein: 1g; Total fat: 2g; Carbohydrates: 1g; Fiber: 1g; Calcium: 10mg; Vitamin D: 0mg; Vitamin B_{12}: 0mg; Iron: 1mg; Zinc: 1mg

MACROS: Protein 7%; Carbs 13%; Fat 80%

VEGAN CAESAR DRESSING

GLUTEN-FREE

LOW-CARB

NUT-FREE

MAKES 1 PINT

PREP TIME: 10 minutes

¾ cup silken tofu

½ cup vegan
   Parmesan cheese

3 tablespoons extra-virgin
   olive oil

3 tablespoons freshly
   squeezed lemon juice

2 teaspoons coarsely
   ground black pepper

Grated zest of 2 lemons

1½ teaspoons
   Dijon mustard

½ teaspoon drained capers

1 large garlic clove

1 teaspoon sea salt, plus
   more as needed

This Caesar dressing is every bit as rich and delicious as the traditional version, but it's 100% plant based and has added protein from the tofu. Use it in a classic Caesar salad with romaine lettuce or kale. It also makes a great veggie dip.

Put the tofu, cheese, oil, lemon juice, pepper, lemon zest, mustard, capers, garlic, and salt in a blender. Puree until smooth. Adjust the seasoning with salt as needed. Use the dressing immediately, or put it in a covered container and refrigerate.

STORAGE: Refrigerate in an airtight container for up to 3 days.

VARIATION: Substitute the flesh of a small, ripe avocado for the tofu, and add 1 teaspoon of chopped jalapeño pepper for a Mexican twist on the classic with added healthy fat.

PER SERVING (2 TABLESPOONS): Calories: 37; Protein: 1g; Total fat: 2g; Carbohydrates: 3g; Fiber: 0g; Calcium: 44mg; Vitamin D: 1mg; Vitamin B$_{12}$: 0mg; Iron: 0mg; Zinc: 0mg

MACROS: Protein 15%; Carbs 31%; Fat 54%

MEDITERRANEAN SPICE BLEND

MAKES ½ CUP

PREP TIME: 5 minutes

¼ cup dried oregano

2 tablespoons
ground cumin

2 tablespoons
smoked paprika

1 tablespoon freshly
ground black pepper

You'll see this spice blend in many recipes throughout the book. Keeping a batch handy will simplify things in the kitchen. It really adds a burst of flavor to just about anything you're cooking. Plus, these spices are also widely used in Latin American and Southeast Asian cooking, so the blend can be used in more than just Mediterranean-inspired dishes.

Put the oregano, cumin, paprika, and pepper in a glass jar, airtight container, or storage bag. Shake vigorously to combine.

STORAGE: This blend will keep in the pantry indefinitely.

COOKING TIP: For extra flavor, toast whole cumin seeds and black peppercorns in a dry skillet over medium-low heat for about 1 minute to release the aromas. Let them cool completely, then grind them to a powder in a spice grinder or blender.

PER SERVING (1 TEASPOON): Calories: 6; Protein: 0g; Total fat: 0g; Carbohydrates: 1g; Fiber: 1g; Calcium: 15mg; Vitamin D: 0mg; Vitamin B_{12}: 0mg; Iron: 1mg; Zinc: 0mg

MACROS: Protein 13%; Carbs 54%; Fat 33%

SPROUTED GRAINS

HIGH-CARB

NUT-FREE

MAKES 2 CUPS

PREP TIME: 5 minutes, plus 2 to 6 days to soak and sprout

½ cup whole grains, such as wheat berries, amaranth, barley, buckwheat, farro, millet, whole oats, quinoa, rice, or rye berries

Water (preferably filtered)

STORAGE: Refrigerate for up to 3 days.

PREP TIP: If you make sprouted grains often, inexpensive sprouting jars made specifically for the purpose can be found online.

Sprouted grains take a little effort and time to make, but they can be worth it for the added protein boost. Sprouting makes some nutrients more bioavailable or absorbable, including protein.

1. Put the grains in a strainer or colander, rinse well with cool water, and drain. Transfer to a small bowl. Cover with water by 2 inches. Let stand at room temperature for at least 12 hours or overnight. Drain through a fine-mesh strainer, rinse well, and drain again.

2. Put the grains in a sterilized 1-quart glass jar and cover with a double layer of cheesecloth secured with a rubber band. Place the jar upside down at an angle in a bowl so that excess water can drain and air can circulate. Keep it out of direct light and ideally at a temperature between 68°F and 75°F.

3. Twice a day, pour water into the jar and swirl it to rinse the grains. Pour off the water and invert the jar again in the bowl as in step 2.

4. Wait and watch: the grains should sprout in 1 to 5 days. They are ready once you see the little sprouts tailing out. You can use them once the sprouts have just emerged or wait until they are longer, about ¼ inch or so.

5. Rinse and drain the sprouted grains before using.

QUINOA PILAF

GLUTEN-FREE

HIGH-CARB

QUENCH THE HUNGER

SERVES 4

PREP TIME: 10 minutes

COOK TIME: 30 minutes

½ cup pine nuts

2 cups red quinoa,
   well rinsed

4½ cups water

½ teaspoon sea salt, plus
   more for seasoning

2 tablespoons extra-virgin
   olive oil

1 teaspoon ground cumin

Grated zest and juice
   of 1 lemon

Freshly ground
   black pepper

1 small red onion,
   finely chopped

½ small bunch fresh
   basil, chopped

2 thyme sprigs, leaves
   stripped off and chopped

STORAGE: Refrigerate
in an airtight container
for up to 5 days. Add
the garnishes when
you are ready to reheat
and serve.

A favorite component for bowls and salads is quinoa, an ancient Peruvian grain containing all nine essential amino acids, making it a complete protein. Serve this pilaf warm with another protein for dinner, or take it along cold as the perfect picnic salad. It can also replace pasta or rice and is wonderful in soup.

1. Put the pine nuts in a small, dry skillet and toast over medium-low heat, tossing frequently to avoid burning, until golden brown. Remove from the heat.

2. In a large saucepan, combine the quinoa, water, and salt. Bring to a boil over medium-high heat.

3. Reduce the heat to medium-low. Cover the saucepan and simmer for about 20 minutes, until the water has been absorbed and the quinoa is tender. Remove from the heat. Transfer to a large bowl. Let sit, covered, for 5 minutes, then fluff with a fork.

4. Stir in the oil, cumin, lemon zest, and lemon juice. Season with salt and pepper.

5. Add the pine nuts, onion, basil, and thyme just before serving.

SERVING TIP: I love this dish in the spring when fresh asparagus rolls around, but it's equally good with green beans, snap peas, or any vegetable you choose.

PER SERVING: Calories: 499; Protein: 15g; Total fat: 24g; Carbohydrates: 60g; Fiber: 7g; Calcium: 59mg; Vitamin D: 0mg; Vitamin B$_{12}$: 0mg; Iron: 5mg; Zinc: 4mg

MACROS: Protein 11%; Carbs 48%; Fat 41%

Tropical Coconut Yogurt Chia Bowls
page 49

3

POWER UP
BREAKFASTS AND SMOOTHIES

A healthy breakfast is essential to start the day off right, yet, for athletes, this meal is easy to skip due to busy schedules or early training sessions. Investing in your morning meal will reap health benefits all day long. Try to eat a meal within one hour of waking up or within one hour of completing a morning training session. This will give your body the fuel it needs for the day and the building blocks to repair muscle tissue. It also helps maintain lean muscle, increase alertness, manage moods, and achieve better blood sugar control throughout the day. These breakfast recipes provide the protein your active body needs, along with wholesome, nourishing ingredients to keep you strong and healthy. You'll find hot and cold options, recipes with only a few ingredients, no-bake recipes, and a few hearty meals worth the extra prep time.

CHERRY BERRY BREAKFAST SMOOTHIE

GLUTEN-FREE

QUENCH THE HUNGER

RECOVERY BOOST

MAKES 1 SMOOTHIE

PREP TIME: 5 minutes

½ cup frozen unsweetened pitted red tart cherries

½ cup frozen blueberries or raspberries (I use a combination)

¼ cup frozen spinach or kale

½ cup unsweetened almond milk or milk of choice

¼ cup 5-Seed Protein Powder (page 19) or store-bought protein powder

¼ cup tart cherry juice

1 tablespoon agave nectar

1 teaspoon coconut oil or MCT oil

½ teaspoon ground cinnamon

Smoothies are a great breakfast choice, because they're fast, portable, nutritious, and easy to digest. This one is my daily go-to. Tart cherries, berries, and greens provide antioxidants that help with inflammation. Adding protein powder and coconut oil rounds this smoothie out into a filling meal.

In a blender, combine the cherries, blueberries, spinach, almond milk, protein powder, cherry juice, agave nectar, oil, and cinnamon. Cover and blend for about 45 seconds, until smooth.

STORAGE: Store in the refrigerator for up to 2 days, or freeze for 1 month. Throw the smoothie in a blender and whip it up again before serving.

SWAP IT: This is a good all-around basic recipe; you can swap out the fruits for any that you like—try mango, pineapple, and coconut milk for a tropical smoothie.

PER SERVING: Calories: 358; Protein: 30g; Total fat: 9g; Carbohydrates: 44g; Fiber: 9g; Calcium: 299mg; Vitamin D: 60mg; Vitamin B$_{12}$: 1mg; Iron: 7mg; Zinc: 3mg

MACROS: Protein 33%; Carbs 45%; Fat 22%

COCONANA BREAKFAST SHAKE

MAKES 1 SHAKE

PREP TIME: 5 minutes

1 frozen banana

½ cup frozen chopped kale
or spinach

½ cup unsweetened
coconut milk

1 scoop (2 tablespoons)
Pea Protein Powder
(page 18) or store-bought
protein powder

1 tablespoon unsweetened
cocoa powder

¼ teaspoon vanilla extract

½ cup ice cubes

1 teaspoon unsweetened
shredded coconut

Pinch ground cinnamon

This is an excellent foundation breakfast smoothie to have in your culinary arsenal, especially for chocolate lovers. Cocoa is a powerful source of antioxidants. As a bonus, it's also rich, delicious, and creates a decadent dessert-like breakfast.

1. In a blender, combine the banana, kale, coconut milk, protein powder, cocoa powder, and vanilla. Blend for about 45 seconds, until smooth.

2. Add the ice cubes as needed for texture, and blend for 15 seconds or until thick and smooth. Pour the shake into a cold glass.

3. Sprinkle with the shredded coconut and cinnamon.

STORAGE: Make a big batch and freeze it in individual resealable bags or containers for up to 2 months. Just pull one out and thaw for a few minutes for a quick breakfast.

SWAP IT: If coconut is not your thing, use any plant-based milk that you prefer; almond or oat milk is also great in this smoothie.

PER SERVING: Calories: 540; Protein: 32g; Total fat: 28g; Carbohydrates: 50g; Fiber: 10g; Calcium: 213mg; Vitamin D: 0mg; Vitamin B_{12}: 0mg; Iron: 12mg; Zinc: 5mg

MACROS: Protein 23%; Carbs 33%; Fat 44%

TROPICAL AVOCADO GREENIE

GLUTEN-FREE
QUENCH THE HUNGER

MAKES 1 GREENIE

PREP TIME: 5 minutes

- ½ ripe avocado, peeled, seeded, and diced, or ¼ cup frozen avocado cubes
- 1 large handful spinach or kale (about 1 cup)
- ½ small cucumber, seeded and diced
- ½ cup pistachios
- ½ cup coconut water or plain water
- ¼ cup unsweetened almond milk or milk of choice
- 1 tablespoon MCT oil
- 6 to 8 fresh mint leaves (optional)
- 1 scoop (2 tablespoons) Pea Protein Powder (page 18) or store-bought protein powder

I have run a few marathons, and although the training is grueling, the reward is well worth it. I developed this smoothie to get me through a long morning run without being hard on my stomach. I still have one of these for breakfast several times a week.

Put the avocado, spinach, cucumber, pistachios, coconut water, almond milk, oil, mint leaves (if using), and protein powder in a blender. Puree for about 1 minute, until very smooth. Serve the smoothie in a tall, cold glass.

PREP AND STORAGE TIP: To save time in the morning, prep the avocado, spinach, banana, cucumber, pineapple, and mint in advance in freezer bags and store in the freezer for up to 6 months. When ready to serve, just pull out a bag, throw it into the blender with the liquids and protein powder, and blend.

PER SERVING: Calories: 682; Protein: 34g; Total fat: 33g; Carbohydrates: 73g; Fiber: 19g; Calcium: 324mg; Vitamin D: 30mg; Vitamin B_{12}: 1mg; Iron: 8mg; Zinc: 5mg

MACROS: Protein 19%; Carbs 40%; Fat 41%

PEANUT BUTTER OVERNIGHT OATS

SERVES 3

PREP TIME: 10 minutes, plus overnight to rest

1½ cups unsweetened
vanilla soy milk or milk
of choice

⅓ cup chia seeds

½ cup peanut butter

1 tablespoon pure
maple syrup

1 teaspoon vanilla extract

¼ teaspoon sea salt

1 cup rolled oats (certified
gluten-free if needed)

Searching for solutions for a rushed morning routine? Look no further than this simple, prep-ahead breakfast; it is nutrient dense, satisfyingly creamy, and delicious. I like to take my oats out of the refrigerator while making coffee so they come to a cool room temperature. You can also enjoy this dish served warm. If you're a peanut butter lover, you might want this meal every day.

1. Put the soy milk, chia seeds, peanut butter, maple syrup, vanilla, and salt in a blender. Blend, starting on low speed and gradually increasing it to high, until smooth.

2. Add the oats and pulse to combine, leaving a little texture. Pour into 3 (8-ounce) glass jars and screw on the jar lids to seal. Refrigerate overnight, and enjoy the next day for breakfast.

STORAGE: Refrigerate in an airtight container for up to 2 days.

VARIATION: For a special breakfast treat, top your oats with a bit of chopped dark chocolate or some chocolate chips.

PER SERVING: Calories: 532; Protein: 21g; Total fat: 34g; Carbohydrates: 45g; Fiber: 13g; Calcium: 341mg; Vitamin D: 0mg; Vitamin B$_{12}$: 1mg; Iron: 4mg; Zinc: 2mg

MACROS: Protein 15%; Carbs 31%; Fat 54%

BLUEBERRY-WALNUT PROTEIN BREAKFAST BARS

GLUTEN-FREE

HIGH-CARB

RECOVERY BOOST

MAKES 12 BARS

PREP TIME: 10 minutes, plus 30 minutes to cool

COOK TIME: 20 minutes

FOR THE PROTEIN BAR BASE

1¾ cups rolled oats

1 cup walnut halves and pieces

½ cup unsweetened applesauce

½ cup 5-Seed Protein Powder (page 19) or store-bought

3 tablespoons pure maple syrup

1 teaspoon vanilla extract

1 teaspoon ground cinnamon

¼ teaspoon sea salt

FOR THE TOPPING

1 cup fresh blueberries

¼ cup rolled oats

¼ cup walnut halves and pieces

¼ cup pumpkin seeds

¼ cup unsweetened soy milk

These next-level crunchy and chewy granola bars are packed with nutrients and antioxidants. They are made with a high-protein base and topped with a blueberry–pumpkin seed crumble. This portable bar will get you going in the morning or keep your energy up as an afternoon snack.

TO MAKE THE PROTEIN BAR BASE

1. Preheat the oven to 350°F. Line a 9-inch square baking pan with parchment paper, leaving 1 inch of extra parchment spilling over the edges of the pan.

2. Put the oats, walnuts, applesauce, protein powder, maple syrup, vanilla, cinnamon, and salt in a food processor or blender. Process until the mixture is thoroughly combined and has formed a smooth dough.

3. Using a spatula, press the dough into the prepared baking pan in an even layer.

4. Transfer the baking pan to the oven and bake for about 8 minutes, until the dough has set.

TO MAKE THE TOPPING

5. Meanwhile, in a medium bowl, combine the blueberries, oats, walnuts, pumpkin seeds, and coconut milk.

6. Remove the baking pan from the oven, and evenly sprinkle the topping mixture over the dough, pressing it in gently.

7. Return the baking pan to the oven and bake for about 12 minutes, until the dough is golden. Remove from the oven. Let cool in the baking dish for 30 minutes, then lift the bars out of the pan with the parchment paper and cut into 12 bars.

STORAGE: Refrigerate in a sealed container for up to 1 week.

VARIATION: The blueberries can be replaced with fresh or dried cranberries, currants, or cherries, or you can make a mixture of your own.

PER SERVING (1 BAR): Calories: 467; Protein: 22g; Total fat: 23g; Carbohydrates: 43g; Fiber: 8g; Calcium: 88mg; Vitamin D: 0mg; Vitamin B$_{12}$: 0mg; Iron: 5mg; Zinc: 5mg

MACROS: Protein 18%; Carbs 36%; Fat 46%

ALMOND YOGURT, FRUIT, AND MUESLI PARFAIT

GLUTEN-FREE
HIGH-CARB
QUENCH THE HUNGER
RECOVERY BOOST

SERVES 3

PREP TIME: 10 minutes, plus 30 minutes to set

COOK TIME: 2 minutes

2 cups rolled oats (certified gluten-free if needed)

½ cup raisins, currants, or your favorite dried fruit

1½ cups unsweetened almond milk

⅓ cup slivered almonds

1¼ cups Almond Milk Yogurt (page 26) or store-bought dairy-free yogurt

4 medium red apples (Macintosh are my favorite), cored and grated

½ cup dried tart cherries, diced

¼ cup freshly squeezed lemon juice

1 tablespoon agave nectar or pure maple syrup

2 cups berries of choice

Mint sprigs, for garnish

True Swiss-style muesli bears little resemblance to the boxed grocery store cereal of the same name. This vegan version is easy to whip up for a healthy breakfast that's sure to fuel your day.

1. In a large bowl, combine the oats and raisins.

2. Add the almond milk, stir to combine, and let sit at room temperature for 30 minutes or until the oats have absorbed all the milk.

3. Meanwhile, heat a small skillet over medium heat.

4. Add the almonds and swirl the skillet to move them around evenly for about 2 minutes, until they turn golden and aromas are released. Remove from the heat. Transfer to a small bowl to cool.

5. To the oat mixture, add the almond yogurt, apples, cherries, lemon juice, and agave nectar. Stir until combined. Spoon into bowls or dessert glasses.

6. Top with the berries and sprinkle with the almonds.

7. Garnish each bowl with a sprig of mint and serve.

STORAGE: Muesli is best eaten right away, but it can be stored in an airtight container in the refrigerator for up to 24 hours.

SWAP IT: Add bananas, coconut milk, dried mango, or pineapple for fun tropical muesli.

PER SERVING: Calories: 781; Protein: 20g; Total fat: 15g; Carbohydrates: 152g; Fiber: 17g; Calcium: 389mg; Vitamin D: 0mg; Vitamin B_{12}: 1mg; Iron: 5mg; Zinc: 4mg

MACROS: Protein 9%; Carbs 75%; Fat 16%

PEANUT BUTTER AND BANANA BREAKFAST COOKIES

MAKES 12 COOKIES

PREP TIME: 5 minutes

COOK TIME: 10 to 15 minutes

2 small ripe bananas
  or 1 large

1 cup rolled oats (certified
  gluten-free if needed)

¼ cup natural peanut
  butter (creamy or
  crunchy)

1 scoop (2 tablespoons)
  Pea Protein Powder
  (page 18) or store-bought
  protein powder

1 tablespoon cocoa powder

¼ teaspoon sea salt

Cookies for breakfast? Yes! These vegan breakfast cookies use only a few ingredients and take about 15 minutes to make. They are a great way to use up overripe bananas. Keep these cookies around for days when you're on the run, or pack them in your gym bag for a postworkout protein snack.

1. Preheat the oven to 350°F. Line a baking sheet with parchment paper.

2. Put the bananas in a medium mixing bowl and mash with a fork.

3. Add the oats, peanut butter, protein powder, cocoa powder, and salt. Stir to thoroughly combine.

4. Scoop 1-inch balls of dough onto the prepared baking sheet. Flatten slightly using the back of a fork.

5. Transfer the baking sheet to the oven and bake for 10 to 12 minutes, until the edges of the cookies are golden brown. Remove from the oven.

STORAGE: The cookies keep for up to 4 days in an airtight container on the counter. Toast them in a toaster oven or warm them in the microwave for a portable breakfast treat.

VARIATION: Add ½ cup of dark chocolate chips, chopped roasted peanuts, or both for an extra-special treat.

PER SERVING (4 COOKIES): Calories: 352; Protein: 20g; Total fat: 12g; Carbohydrates: 44g; Fiber: 8g; Calcium: 56mg; Vitamin D: 0mg; Vitamin B$_{12}$: 0mg; Iron: 4mg; Zinc: 4mg

MACROS: Protein 22%; Carbs 48%; Fat 30%

SEITAN BREAKFAST BURRITOS

QUENCH THE HUNGER
RECOVERY BOOST

MAKES 4 BURRITOS

PREP TIME: 15 minutes
COOK TIME: 20 minutes

1 tablespoon avocado oil

1 small yellow onion, diced

2 garlic cloves, minced

Sea salt

8 ounces Basic Seitan (page 20) or store-bought, diced

1 small jalapeño pepper, seeded and minced

2 ripe plum tomatoes, diced

2 teaspoons Mediterranean Spice Blend (page 30)

1 (15-ounce) can kidney beans (or any variety), drained and rinsed

4 (10-inch) corn tortillas

1 ripe avocado, pitted, peeled, and sliced

¼ small head red cabbage, cored and thinly sliced

½ cup crumbled Vegan Soft Cheese (page 24) or store-bought

Tired of oatmeal for breakfast? These savory, plant-based breakfast burritos are sure to break up any breakfast boredom.

1. In a medium skillet, heat the oil over medium-high heat until it begins to shimmer.

2. Add the onion and sauté for 3 to 4 minutes, until translucent. Add the garlic and salt. Cook for 1 minute.

3. Reduce the heat to medium. Add the seitan, jalapeño, and tomatoes. Sauté for 5 minutes.

4. Add the spice blend and cook for 1 to 2 minutes. Add the beans and stir to combine. Cook for about 4 minutes, until heated through. Remove from the heat. Cover to keep warm.

5. To warm the tortillas, place them between a layer of paper towels and microwave for 1 minute.

6. Lay the tortillas out on a clean surface. Place about 2 to 3 tablespoons each of the vegetable and bean mixture, avocado, and cabbage onto each tortilla.

7. Sprinkle the cheese on top, and roll up the burritos tightly. Serve.

STORAGE: Refrigerate for up to 4 days, or freeze for up to 2 months.

PER SERVING (1 BURRITO): Calories: 491; Protein: 33g; Total fat: 19g; Carbohydrates: 47g; Fiber: 12g; Calcium: 227mg; Vitamin D: 0mg; Vitamin B_{12}: 0mg; Iron: 5mg; Zinc: 2mg

MACROS: Protein 27%; Carbs 38%; Fat 35%

TOFU HUMMUS AND SPROUTED GRAIN SOURDOUGH TOAST

HIGH-CARB

NUT-FREE

RECOVERY BOOST

MAKES 4 TOASTS

PREP TIME: 15 minutes

COOK TIME: 5 minutes

FOR THE TOFU HUMMUS

1 pound fresh tofu (page 22) or store-bought silken tofu

2 tablespoons tahini

1 tablespoon extra-virgin olive oil

4 garlic cloves, crushed

1 tablespoon freshly squeezed lemon juice

1 teaspoon sea salt, plus more as needed

Freshly ground black pepper

FOR THE TOASTS

4 sprouted sourdough bread slices, toasted

2 ripe avocados, pitted, peeled, and sliced

4 ounces Sprouted Grains (page 31) or salad sprouts such as alfalfa or pea

1 teaspoon smoked paprika

Although traditional hummus is a great vegan snack, this tofu version is packed with protein, and it's a snap to whip up for breakfast. Spread it on your favorite bread, bagel, or sprouted sourdough bread—as in this version—for an extra protein kick.

TO MAKE THE TOFU HUMMUS

1. Put the tofu, tahini, oil, and garlic in a food processor. Process until smooth.

2. Add the lemon juice and salt, and process until smooth. Adjust the seasoning with salt and pepper as needed.

TO MAKE THE TOASTS

3. Spread the hummus on the toasts.

4. Top with the avocado and sprinkle with the sprouted grains and paprika. Serve immediately.

STORAGE: This is best served immediately, but the hummus will keep for up to 7 days in an airtight container in the refrigerator.

SERVING TIP: This can be packed with crackers or raw vegetables for a great on-the-go snack.

PER SERVING (1 TOAST): Calories: 492; Protein: 20g; Total fat: 28g; Carbohydrates: 47g; Fiber: 10g; Calcium: 220mg; Vitamin D: 0mg; Vitamin B$_{12}$: 0mg; Iron: 5mg; Zinc: 2mg

MACROS: Protein 16%; Carbs 36%; Fat 48%

TOFU AND CHORIZO BREAKFAST TACOS

SERVES 3

PREP TIME: 20 minutes

COOK TIME: 20 minutes

½ tablespoon olive oil

1 small jalapeño pepper,
seeded and diced

½ medium red onion, diced

3 plum tomatoes

1 tablespoon
smoked paprika

1 teaspoon sea salt, plus
more as needed

½ teaspoon ground cumin

¼ teaspoon ground
turmeric

1 (16-ounce) package firm
tofu, drained and rinsed

4 ounces vegan chorizo,
cooked and crumbled

Juice of 1 lime (optional)

12 (4-inch) corn tortillas

Salsa, for serving

To get the best texture in a tofu scramble, you must press out as much water as possible from the tofu. Once your tofu is drained, press it in a tofu press or under a cast-iron skillet for 5 to 10 minutes. These protein-packed power tacos can fuel a tough morning of work or your workouts.

1. In a large skillet, heat the oil over medium heat.

2. Add the jalapeño and onion. Sauté for 4 to 5 minutes, until softened.

3. Meanwhile, put the tomatoes in a blender and pulse a few times. The tomatoes should be thoroughly chopped but still have a bit of texture.

4. To the jalapeño and onion mixture, add the paprika, salt, cumin, and turmeric. Sauté for 1 minute or until the spice aromas are released.

5. Stir in the tomatoes and crumble in the tofu. Simmer for 10 minutes, stirring occasionally, or until the liquid reduces.

6. Stir in the chorizo and lime juice (if using). Simmer, stirring constantly, for 1 minute. Remove from the heat.

7. To warm the tortillas, place them between layers of paper towels and microwave for 1 minute.

8. Taste the filling and adjust the seasoning with more salt if needed. Fold the filling inside the warm tortillas with your favorite salsa, and serve immediately.

STORAGE: Refrigerate the filling and tortillas separately in airtight containers for up to 5 days.

INGREDIENT TIP: If you have easy access to an Indian grocery store or gourmet market, Himalayan black salt makes tofu taste exactly like scrambled eggs.

PER SERVING: Calories: 328; Protein: 20g; Total fat: 15g; Carbohydrates: 34g; Fiber: 6g; Calcium: 323mg; Vitamin D: 0mg; Vitamin B$_{12}$: 0mg; Iron: 5mg; Zinc: 2mg

MACROS: Protein 21%; Carbs 40%; Fat 39%

POWER PANCAKES

GLUTEN-FREE
LOW-CARB
NUT-FREE
QUENCH THE HUNGER

When I'm craving something heartier for break-fast, these pancakes are the perfect fit. They're homey and comforting and can be made almost as quickly as whipping up a smoothie.

SERVES 1

PREP TIME: 15 minutes
COOK TIME: 10 minutes

2 tablespoons ground flaxseed or ground chia seeds
5 tablespoons water
2 scoops (¼ cup) 5-Seed Protein Powder (page 19) or store-bought vanilla protein powder
1 large very ripe banana
¼ teaspoon baking powder
¼ teaspoon sea salt
⅛ teaspoon ground cinnamon
Fresh fruit, for serving

1. In a small bowl, stir together the flaxseed and water. Set aside for about 10 minutes. The mixture will thicken to become flax eggs.

2. In a medium bowl, combine the protein powder, banana, baking powder, salt, and cinnamon. Using a whisk or an electric hand beater, beat until smooth.

3. Fold in the flax eggs until well combined.

4. Heat a medium nonstick skillet over low heat.

5. Scoop ¼ cup of the batter onto the skillet and cook for about 1 minute per side, until golden brown. Repeat with the remaining batter. Remove from the heat.

6. Serve the pancakes warm with fresh fruit.

STORAGE: This is a great recipe to double and store for meal prepping. The pancakes keep in the refrigerator for 3 days or in the freezer for 3 months.

VARIATION: For a luxurious topping, mix a little Almond Milk Yogurt (page 26), your favorite berries, and a touch of maple syrup.

PER SERVING (4 PANCAKES): Calories: 282; Protein: 22g; Total fat: 6g; Carbohydrates: 38g; Fiber: 8g; Calcium: 216mg; Vitamin D: 0mg; Vitamin B$_{12}$: 0mg; Iron: 2mg; Zinc: 2mg

MACROS: Protein 32%; Carbs 48%; Fat 20%

TROPICAL COCONUT YOGURT CHIA BOWLS

GLUTEN-FREE
NUT-FREE
QUENCH THE HUNGER
RECOVERY BOOST

SERVES 2

PREP TIME: 5 minutes, plus overnight to rest

2 cups coconut milk yogurt

½ cup unsweetened coconut milk

1 scoop (2 tablespoons) Pea Protein Powder (page 18) or store-bought protein powder

2 tablespoons chia seeds

1 banana

½ cup diced pineapple fresh or dried

½ cup diced mango fresh or dried

2 tablespoons unsweetened coconut flakes, lightly toasted

1 tablespoon sesame seeds, lightly toasted

Chia is one of my favorite nutrition powerhouses, mainly because it's so versatile. You can put it in anything and reap the benefits of its omega-3 fatty acids and antioxidants. This bowl combines chia seeds with coconut milk yogurt for a creamy breakfast pudding. If you don't have fresh fruit on hand, use dried. You can also swap the sesame seeds for chopped nuts, such as pistachios.

1. Put the coconut milk yogurt, coconut milk, protein powder, and chia seeds in a medium glass mixing bowl. Whisk to combine thoroughly. Cover and refrigerate overnight.

2. When ready to serve, transfer the yogurt mixture to individual serving bowls.

3. Arrange the banana, pineapple, and mango on top.

4. Sprinkle with the coconut flakes and sesame seeds.

STORAGE: Refrigerate in a sealed container for up to 3 days.

COOKING TIP: Toast the coconut and sesame seeds separately in a small dry skillet over medium-low heat, tossing frequently to avoid burning, until golden brown.

PER SERVING: Calories: 655; Protein: 27g; Total fat: 27g; Carbohydrates: 82g; Fiber: 11g; Calcium: 465mg; Vitamin D: 0mg; Vitamin B$_{12}$: 0mg; Iron: 9mg; Zinc: 4mg

MACROS: Protein 16%; Carbs 35%; Fat 49%

BREAKFAST QUINOA WITH CHAI-SPICED WALNUTS

GLUTEN-FREE

HIGH-CARB

QUENCH THE HUNGER

SERVES 2

PREP TIME: 15 minutes, plus overnight to soak

COOK TIME: 25 minutes

FOR THE CHAI-SPICED WALNUTS

3 tablespoons pure maple syrup

2 tablespoons extra-virgin olive oil

2½ teaspoons chai spice blend

3 cups walnut halves and pieces

FOR THE QUINOA

3 cups water, divided

½ cup quinoa

2 tablespoons millet

2 tablespoons ground flaxseed

1 tablespoon pure maple syrup

1 teaspoon sea salt

½ teaspoon ground cinnamon

¼ teaspoon ground nutmeg

¼ teaspoon ground cloves

There are few things more comforting than a bowl of hot cereal on a cold morning. Instead of the usual, try this protein-rich quinoa version with a touch of maple syrup for a special winter breakfast packed with nutrients.

TO MAKE THE CHAI-SPICED WALNUTS

1. Preheat the oven to 325°F. Line a baking sheet with parchment paper.

2. In a medium bowl, whisk together the maple syrup, oil, and spice blend.

3. Add the walnuts and toss until well coated.

4. Spread the nuts out in an even layer on the prepared baking sheet.

5. Transfer the baking sheet to the oven and roast for 15 to 20 minutes, stirring every 5 minutes, until the nuts are golden and fragrant. Remove from the oven. Let cool and transfer to a sealed container until you're ready to use them.

TO MAKE THE QUINOA

6. In a medium saucepan, combine 1½ cups of water, the quinoa, millet, and flaxseed. Cover and soak at room temperature overnight.

7. In the morning, heat the saucepan with the soaked grains over medium heat.

8. Add the remaining 1½ cups of water, the maple syrup, salt, cinnamon, nutmeg, and cloves. Simmer for about 5 minutes, stirring occasionally, until the grains become soft and the mixture thickens. Remove from the heat.

9. Serve the quinoa warm, topped with the walnuts.

STORAGE: Store the nuts for about 1 week in an airtight container on the countertop. Refrigerate the quinoa separately for up to 1 week.

SWAP IT: You can use any of your favorite whole grains, as long as the ratio is 3:1 water to grains. I use my favorite mix here, but feel free to make it your own; the method is the same.

PER SERVING (WITH ½ CUP WALNUT HALVES AS TOPPING): Calories: 1120; Protein: 24g; Total fat: 86g; Carbohydrates: 72g; Fiber: 14g; Calcium: 198mg; Vitamin D: 0mg; Vitamin B$_{12}$: 0mg; Iron: 6mg; Zinc: 6mg

MACROS: Protein 8%; Carbs 27%; Fat 65%

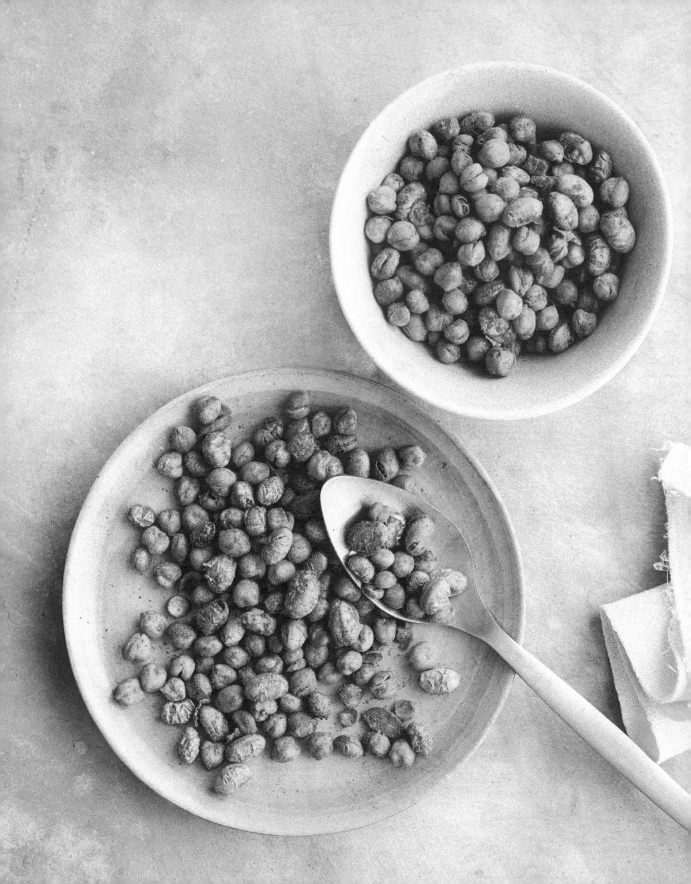

PORTABLE PROTEIN SNACKS

4

Let's face it: snacks can get monotonous. This is especially true when trying to choose high-protein vegan snacks. Snack time is a crucial opportunity for athletes to meet their protein needs. Have no fear; this chapter is here to help. In this chapter, you will find all kinds of portable snacks that are far from boring. Familiar flavors are used in whole new applications to keep high-protein snacking doable and interesting.

Crispy Cinnamon Chickpeas
page 56

EASY PEANUT BUTTER PROTEIN BARS

MAKES 9 BARS

PREP TIME: 10 minutes, plus 30 minutes to chill

¾ cup creamy natural peanut butter

¼ cup agave nectar

1 tablespoon melted coconut oil

1 teaspoon vanilla extract

¼ cup ground flaxseed

½ cup 5-Seed Protein Powder (page 19) or store-bought protein powder

3 ounces dairy-free dark chocolate, chopped

Sea salt, for sprinkling

INGREDIENT TIP: Real dark chocolate does not contain dairy, but some large manufacturers use dairy products in their chocolate. Check the label.

I developed this no-bake protein bar recipe for a low-carb, high-protein snack that keeps me energized and satisfies my sweet tooth. This is a perfect snack to eat 1 to 2 hours before a workout or to refuel with afterward.

1. Line an 8-inch square baking dish with parchment paper.

2. To make the batter, in a medium bowl, using a firm whisk or fork, whisk together the peanut butter, agave nectar, oil, and vanilla until smooth.

3. Add the flaxseed and protein powder. Stir to combine. Using your hands, work the batter into a cookie dough texture. Press the dough into the prepared baking dish.

4. In a small saucepan, melt the chocolate over low heat until completely smooth. Remove from the heat.

5. Pour the chocolate evenly over the dough, and tilt and swirl the dish to make an even layer. Sprinkle with salt. Refrigerate for at least 30 minutes to allow the bars to set. Cut into 9 bars or squares, cover, and refrigerate until ready to eat.

STORAGE: Refrigerate in an airtight container for up to 1 week, or freeze for 3 months.

PER SERVING (1 BAR): Calories: 284; Protein: 16g; Total fat: 18g; Carbohydrates: 16g; Fiber: 5g; Calcium: 156mg; Vitamin D: 0mg; Vitamin B$_{12}$: 0mg; Iron: 4mg; Zinc: 2mg

MACROS: Protein 22%; Carbs 55%; Fat 23%

LEMON-COCONUT PROTEIN BALLS

MAKES 12 BALLS

PREP TIME: 10 minutes, plus 30 minutes to set

1 cup raw cashews

1 cup rolled oats (certified gluten-free if needed)

1 cup unsweetened desiccated coconut, divided (see headnote)

1 tablespoon coconut oil

Pinch sea salt

½ cup 5-Seed Protein Powder (page 19) or store-bought protein powder

Grated zest and juice of 1 medium lemon

¼ cup agave nectar

VARIATION: These are amazing made with any kind of citrus; try using pink grapefruit or tangerine.

Toss these zesty lemon balls in your gym bag for a portable pre-or postworkout treat. They are also excellent as an afternoon snack or even a quick breakfast in a pinch. Desiccated coconut is dried and finely ground. If you can't find it, use finely ground almonds or pistachios as a great alternative.

1. Put the cashews, oats, ⅔ cup of desiccated coconut, the oil, and salt in a food processor. Process for about 2 minutes, until fine.

2. Add the protein powder and lemon zest. Pulse until well combined.

3. Add the agave nectar, then slowly add the lemon juice in a thin stream, pulsing until the mixture has a firm but sticky texture.

4. Spread the remaining ⅓ cup of desiccated coconut on a large plate.

5. Scoop the mixture into 12 individual balls, roll between your hands until smooth, and then roll each in the coconut to coat evenly. Refrigerate until firm, about 30 minutes, before eating.

STORAGE: Refrigerate in an airtight container for up to 1 week.

PER SERVING (2 BALLS): Calories: 342; Protein: 19g; Total fat: 20g; Carbohydrates: 26g; Fiber: 6g; Calcium: 112mg; Vitamin D: 0mg; Vitamin B$_{12}$: 0mg; Iron: 6mg; Zinc: 4mg

MACROS: Protein 19%; Carbs 32%; Fat 49%

CRISPY CINNAMON CHICKPEAS

GLUTEN-FREE

LOW-CARB

NUT-FREE

RECOVERY BOOST

These crispy, crunchy little bites are quick and easy to make with very few ingredients. They are irresistible for snacking and a great protein-packed topping for salads or bowls. For a variation, try half chickpeas and half edamame.

SERVES 4

PREP TIME: 10 minutes, plus 30 minutes to dry

COOK TIME: 45 minutes

2 (15-ounce) cans chickpeas, drained and rinsed

2 tablespoons olive oil

2 tablespoons za'atar spice blend (see tip)

2 tablespoons ground cinnamon

1 teaspoon pure maple syrup

½ teaspoon smoked paprika

1 teaspoon sea salt

1. Preheat the oven to 400°F.

2. Spread the chickpeas out on a baking sheet to air-dry for at least 30 minutes; the drier the chickpeas, the crispier they will be when baked.

3. In a medium bowl, whisk together the oil, za'atar, cinnamon, maple syrup, paprika, and salt.

4. Add the chickpeas and toss to coat.

5. Line a baking sheet with parchment paper. Spread the chickpeas out in a single layer.

6. Transfer the baking sheet to the oven; bake for 45 minutes or until the chickpeas are golden brown and crunchy. Remove from the oven.

STORAGE TIP: Store in an airtight container at room temperature for up to 1 week; recrisp in the oven at 350°F for 10 minutes as needed.

INGREDIENT TIP: Za'atar is a common Mediterranean spice blend that includes sesame seeds, sumac, thyme, and oregano. If you can't find it, use Mediterranean Spice Blend (page 30), garam masala, or curry powder.

PER SERVING: Calories: 276; Protein: 11g; Total fat: 10g; Carbohydrates: 38g; Fiber: 12g; Calcium: 102mg; Vitamin D: 0mg; Vitamin B$_{12}$: 0mg; Iron: 4mg; Zinc: 2mg

MACROS: Protein 14%; Carbs 54%; Fat 32%

POWER TRAIL MIX

MAKES 3 POUNDS

PREP TIME: 5 minutes

COOK TIME: 15 minutes

¾ cup raw walnut pieces

¾ cup raw cashews

½ cup raw sunflower seeds

½ cup raw pumpkin seeds

¼ cup ground flaxseed

½ cup dried tart cherries

½ cup raisins

½ cup chopped dairy-free
dark chocolate

½ teaspoon
ground cinnamon

¼ teaspoon sea salt

STORAGE: Store in an airtight container on the counter for up to 1 month.

When you're an athlete, a stash of emergency snacks makes it easier to stay on track with healthy, plant-rich eating. This chocolate, seed, and fruit trail mix is an ideal choice. Besides being delicious, dark chocolate is a powerful source of antioxidants and a natural energy lifter! Look for unsulfured dried fruits, because sulfured are treated with a chemical preservative.

1. Preheat the oven to 350°F. Line a baking sheet with parchment paper.

2. In a medium bowl, toss together the walnuts, cashews, sunflower seeds, pumpkin seeds, and flaxseed until combined.

3. Spread the mixture out on the prepared baking sheet.

4. Transfer the baking sheet to the oven and toast for 10 to 15 minutes, until the mixture is golden. Remove from the oven. Set aside to cool.

5. In a large bowl, combine the cherries, raisins, chocolate, cinnamon, and salt. Mix well.

6. Mix in the cooled nuts.

SWAP IT: Use your favorite combination of fruits and nuts; dried apricots, bananas, and cranberries are great choices.

PER SERVING (¾ CUP): Calories: 253; Protein: 7g; Total fat: 18g; Carbohydrates: 19g; Fiber: 4g; Calcium: 38mg; Vitamin D: 0mg; Vitamin B_{12}: 0mg; Iron: 3mg; Zinc: 2mg

MACROS: Protein 10%; Carbs 28%; Fat 62%

PROTEIN BROWNIE BITES

GLUTEN-FREE
HIGH-CARB
QUENCH THE HUNGER
RECOVERY BOOST

MAKES 12 BROWNIES

PREP TIME: 5 minutes

COOK TIME: 15 minutes, plus 30 minutes to chill

Nonstick cooking spray

1 cup mashed over-ripe bananas (about 2 bananas)

½ cup almond butter or any nut butter

½ cup Dutch-process cocoa powder

2 scoops (¼ cup) 5-Seed Protein Powder (page 19) or store-bought protein powder

Pinch sea salt

1 tablespoon coconut sugar, or sweetener of choice

STORAGE: Store the brownies in an airtight container in the refrigerator for up to 1 week; they can also be frozen for 6 months.

Turn brownies into a super snack with this easy recipe. This vegan, flourless version is protein packed, thanks to the protein powder and nut butter. They're also paleo friendly and low carb. If you don't like bananas, try using pumpkin or sweet potato puree instead.

1. Preheat the oven to 350°F. Grease a mini muffin tin, then line it with 12 liners, or grease an 8-inch square baking pan and line it with parchment paper.

2. In a high-speed blender or food processor, combine the bananas, almond butter, cocoa powder, protein powder, and salt. Blend or process until smooth.

3. Pour the brownie mixture into the prepared muffin cups or baking pan.

4. Sprinkle with the coconut sugar.

5. Transfer to the oven; bake for 10 to 12 minutes, until a cake tester or toothpick comes out clean. Remove from the oven. Let cool completely in the pan on a cooling rack. Once cooled, refrigerate for 30 minutes before serving to allow the bites to set.

SWAP IT: For nut-free brownies, use sunflower seed butter or tahini.

PER SERVING (2 BROWNIES): Calories: 244; Protein: 14g; Total fat: 14g; Carbohydrates: 24g; Fiber: 6g; Calcium: 110mg; Vitamin D: 0mg; Vitamin B$_{12}$: 0mg; Iron: 4mg; Zinc: 2mg

MACROS: Protein 21%; Carbs 33%; Fat 46%

ROASTED EDAMAME

GLUTEN-FREE
LOW-CARB
NUT-FREE
RECOVERY BOOST

SERVES 3

PREP TIME: 5 minutes
COOK TIME: 15 minutes

1 tablespoon olive oil
½ teaspoon chili powder
¼ teaspoon dried basil
¼ teaspoon garlic powder
¼ teaspoon ground cumin
¼ teaspoon
  smoked paprika
¼ teaspoon sea salt
¼ teaspoon freshly ground
  black pepper
1 (12-ounce) package
  shelled edamame
  (thawed and patted dry
  if frozen)

Need something crispy and salty that'll fill you up and keep you satisfied until there's time for a meal? Roasted edamame is a protein-rich, powerhouse snack that will satisfy cravings to help you refuel after a workout.

1. Preheat the oven to 375°F. Line a baking sheet with parchment paper.

2. In a mixing bowl, whisk together the oil, chili powder, basil, garlic powder, cumin, paprika, salt, and pepper.

3. Add the edamame and stir to coat well.

4. Spread the edamame out in a single layer on the prepared baking sheet.

5. Transfer the baking sheet to the oven and roast for 12 to 15 minutes, stirring halfway through, until the edamame begin to turn golden. Remove from the oven. Let cool for 5 minutes on the baking sheet.

STORAGE: Refrigerate in a sealed container for up to 5 days; crisp up any leftovers in a 350°F oven for 10 minutes before serving.

VARIATION: Roasted edamame can also be served hot as a side dish or as a bowl component. Use any spice blend you like for variety, or add some cayenne for a spicy kick.

PER SERVING: Calories: 278; Protein: 21g; Total fat: 14g; Carbohydrates: 20g; Fiber: 10g; Calcium: 126mg; Vitamin D: 0mg; Vitamin B$_{12}$: 0mg; Iron: 5mg; Zinc: 3mg

MACROS: Protein 26%; Carbs 29%; Fat 45%

ICED COFFEE PROTEIN SHAKE

GLUTEN-FREE
LOW-CARB
RECOVERY BOOST

MAKES 2 SHAKES

PREP TIME: 5 minutes

1 cup cold brewed coffee
   (or 1 tablespoon instant
   espresso powder and
   1 cup water)
½ cup unsweetened
   almond milk or dairy-free
   milk of choice
1 scoop (2 tablespoons)
   Pea Protein Powder
   (page 18) or store-bought
   protein powder
2 tablespoons ground
   hemp seeds or flaxseed
½ teaspoon pure
   maple syrup
½ teaspoon vanilla extract
2 cups ice cubes

If you want more than caffeine from your coffee, turn it into this rich and delicious shake. It's inspired by my favorite coffee ice cream—indulgent in flavor but without added sugar. The protein and healthy fat will keep you energized long after the caffeine buzz wears off.

Put the coffee, almond milk, protein powder, ground hemp seeds, maple syrup, vanilla, and ice in a high-speed blender. Blend until smooth and creamy. Pour the shake into cold glasses and enjoy immediately.

STORAGE: This is best served fresh to maintain a luscious texture.

VARIATION: For an extra-special treat, freeze this shake in ice cube trays, then use the cubes to ice your coffee.

PER SERVING (1 SHAKE): Calories: 153; Protein: 16g; Total fat: 5g; Carbohydrates: 11g; Fiber: 4g; Calcium: 137mg; Vitamin D: 0mg; Vitamin B$_{12}$: 1mg; Iron: 3mg; Zinc: 2mg

MACROS: Protein 41%; Carbs 29%; Fat 30%

BANANA-WALNUT POWER BREAD

HIGH-CARB

QUENCH THE HUNGER

SERVES 8

PREP TIME: 10 minutes, plus 10 minutes to soak

COOK TIME: 45 to 50 minutes, plus 10 minutes to cool

2 tablespoons ground chia seeds or flaxseed

5 tablespoons water

1 cup all-purpose flour

½ cup Pea Protein Powder (page 18) or store-bought protein powder

1 teaspoon baking powder

1 teaspoon baking soda

1 teaspoon ground cinnamon

¾ teaspoon sea salt

4 medium over-ripe bananas

½ cup coconut sugar or sweetener of choice

¼ cup agave nectar

⅓ cup avocado oil

1 teaspoon vanilla extract

½ cup walnuts, chopped

½ cup vegan dark chocolate chips

This vegan banana bread is easy to make with on-hand pantry ingredients. It's also a great use of overripe bananas.

1. Preheat the oven to 350°F. Line a 9-by-5-inch loaf pan with parchment paper.

2. In a small bowl, stir together the ground chia seeds and water. Set aside for about 10 minutes. The mixture will thicken to become flax eggs.

3. In a medium bowl, whisk together the flour, protein powder, baking powder, baking soda, cinnamon, and salt.

4. In a large bowl, mash the bananas with a fork. Add the chia eggs, sugar, agave nectar, oil, and vanilla; whisk to combine.

5. Add the flour mixture to the banana mixture, and use a spatula to fold the ingredients together until just combined; the batter will be very thick. Gently fold in the walnuts.

6. Pour the mixture into the prepared loaf pan and sprinkle with the chocolate chips.

7. Transfer the loaf pan to the oven and bake for 45 to 50 minutes, until a toothpick comes out clean. Remove from the oven. Let the loaf cool for 10 minutes before transferring it to a cooling rack. Let cool completely, then slice.

PER SERVING: Calories: 380; Protein: 9g; Total fat: 19g; Carbohydrates: 46g; Fiber: 5g; Calcium: 105mg; Vitamin D: 0mg; Vitamin B$_{12}$: 0mg; Iron: 2mg; Zinc: 1mg

MACROS: Protein 10%; Carbs 46%; Fat 44%

OVERNIGHT OAT AND DRIED CHERRY COOKIES

HIGH-CARB

QUENCH THE HUNGER

RECOVERY BOOST

MAKES 24 COOKIES

PREP TIME: 20 minutes, plus at least 6 hours to soak

COOK TIME: 15 minutes

2 tablespoons ground flax-seed or chia seeds

5 tablespoons water

1 cup vegan butter, softened

1 cup coconut sugar, or sweetener of choice

½ cup plus

1 tablespoon pure maple syrup, divided

2 teaspoons vanilla extract

1 cup all-purpose flour

¼ cup Pea Protein Powder (page 18) or store-bought protein powder

1 teaspoon ground cinnamon

1 teaspoon baking soda

1 teaspoon sea salt

3 cups rolled oats

½ cup chopped pecans

½ cup dried tart cherries, chopped

2 tablespoons toasted pumpkin seeds

Oats are an awesome snack choice for athletes, but oatmeal can get monotonous and is difficult to eat on the go. These cookies were a happy accident, created by leaving overnight oats on the kitchen counter all day, where they dried into a cookie texture. That batch was far from perfect, but through trial and error, I came up with this moist, chewy treat.

1. In a small bowl, stir together the ground flaxseed and water. Set aside for about 10 minutes. The mixture will thicken to become flax eggs.

2. Put the vegan butter in the bowl of a stand mixer fitted with the paddle attachment (or a large bowl, if using a hand mixer).

3. Add the coconut sugar and ½ cup maple syrup. Beat on high speed for about 4 minutes, until the mixture is light and fluffy.

4. Beat in the flax eggs, and scrape down the sides of the bowl. Turn off the mixer.

5. Fold in the remaining tablespoon maple syrup and vanilla until just combined.

6. In a medium bowl, whisk together the flour, protein powder, cinnamon, baking soda, and salt.

7. Gradually add the flour mixture to the mixer, and beat on low speed for about 2 minutes, until combined.

8. Fold in the oats, pecans, cherries, and pumpkin seeds. Stir to combine. Cover the bowl tightly with plastic wrap and refrigerate for at least 6 hours or overnight.

9. Preheat the oven to 350°F. Line 2 baking sheets with parchment paper.

10. Scoop out 24 balls of batter, about 2 tablespoons each, and place them on the prepared baking sheets.

11. Transfer the baking sheets to the oven and bake for 12 to 14 minutes, until the edges begin to turn golden brown. Remove from the oven.

STORAGE: Store in a sealed container at room temperature for up to 5 days, or refrigerate for up to 2 weeks.

VARIATION: This recipe is perfect for improvising. Add your favorite dried fruits, nuts, seeds, or candy chips.

PER SERVING (2 COOKIES): Calories: 424; Protein: 10g; Total fat: 22g; Carbohydrates: 50g; Fiber: 4g; Calcium: 70mg; Vitamin D: 0mg; Vitamin B_{12}: 0mg; Iron: 2mg; Zinc: 2mg

MACROS: Protein 8%; Carbs 48%; Fat 44%

CARROT CAKE PROTEIN BALLS

MAKES 24 BALLS

PREP TIME: 10 minutes, plus 30 minutes to chill

2 medium carrots, peeled and finely grated

1 cup peanut butter or any nut butter

1 cup rolled oats (certified gluten-free if needed)

½ cup unsweetened shredded coconut

½ cup Pea Protein Powder (page 18) or store-bought protein powder

2 tablespoons ground flaxseed

½ cup pure maple syrup

½ teaspoon vanilla extract

1 teaspoon ground cinnamon

¼ teaspoon ground allspice

¼ teaspoon sea salt

Need a simple solution for the dreaded afternoon slump? These tempting protein balls are a real treat and have healthy fats, whole grains, and, of course, ample protein. They are a great addition to your gym bag snack rotation.

1. Line a baking sheet with parchment paper.

2. Put the carrots, peanut butter, oats, coconut, protein powder, flaxseed, maple syrup, vanilla, cinnamon, allspice, and salt in a stand mixer fitted with a paddle attachment (or a large bowl, if using a hand mixer). Mix on medium speed for about 3 minutes, until well combined.

3. Scrape down the sides of the bowl, then mix again for 1 minute. Turn off the mixer.

4. Using a 1-ounce scoop or large soup spoon, portion the dough into 24 small balls, and place them on the prepared baking sheet. Refrigerate for 30 minutes.

5. Roll the balls until they are smooth and round.

STORAGE: Refrigerate in an airtight container for up to 5 days.

VARIATION: Dip these in a little cream cheese frosting for a dessert treat.

PER SERVING (2 BALLS): Calories: 270; Protein: 14g; Total fat: 14g; Carbohydrates: 24g; Fiber: 4g; Calcium: 126mg; Vitamin D: 0mg; Vitamin B$_{12}$: 0mg; Iron: 4mg; Zinc: 2mg

MACROS: Protein 20%; Carbs 35%; Fat 45%

BANANA, CACAO, AND COCONUT SMOOTHIE

GLUTEN-FREE

RECOVERY BOOST

MAKES 2 SMOOTHIES

PREP TIME: 10 minutes

This is as close as you can get to a healthy milk-shake! The smoothie is a tempting concoction of frozen banana, shredded coconut, dates, cacao powder, almond butter, and almond milk. If you don't have cacao, feel free to sub in cocoa powder.

FOR THE CACAO SAUCE

2 tablespoons
   cacao powder

2 tablespoons coconut
   oil, melted

2 tablespoons pure
   maple syrup

¼ teaspoon vanilla extract

¼ teaspoon sea salt

FOR THE SMOOTHIE

2 medium frozen
   bananas, sliced

2 tablespoons unsweet-
   ened shredded coconut

2 pitted medjool dates

1 tablespoon cacao powder

1 tablespoon almond butter

1 scoop (2 tablespoons)
   5-Seed Protein Powder
   (page 19) or store-bought

1 cup unsweetened vanilla
   almond milk

> **VARIATION:** Add
> 2 tablespoons
> old-fashioned oats for a
> thicker shake.

TO MAKE THE CACAO SAUCE

1. In a small bowl, whisk together the cacao powder, oil, maple syrup, vanilla, and salt for about 2 minutes, until smooth and completely combined.

TO MAKE THE SMOOTHIE

2. Put the bananas, coconut, dates, cacao powder, almond butter, protein powder, and almond milk in a high-speed blender. Blend on high speed until smooth and creamy.

3. Swirl the cacao sauce in rings inside 2 large glasses or resealable pint jars.

4. Pour the smoothie in the glasses, and top with an extra drizzle of cacao sauce.

STORAGE: The cacao sauce will hold well in the refrigerator for up to 1 week. Pop it into the microwave for a few seconds to loosen it up before using. Store the smoothie for up to 3 days in an airtight container in the refrigerator.

PER SERVING (1 SMOOTHIE): Calories: 554; Protein: 21g; Total fat: 24g; Carbohydrates: 74g; Fiber: 10g; Calcium: 269mg; Vitamin D: 0mg; Vitamin B_{12}: 1mg; Iron: 5mg, Zinc: 3mg

MACROS: Protein 14%; Carbs 48%; Fat 38%

MANGO-CHIA RECOVERY SHAKE

GLUTEN-FREE

HIGH-CARB

NUT-FREE

RECOVERY BOOST

MAKES 2 SMOOTHIES

PREP TIME: 15 minutes

2 tablespoons chia seeds

1½ cups unsweetened soy
milk or dairy-free milk of
choice, divided

1 medium frozen
banana, sliced

2 cups frozen
mango chunks

1 cup frozen pine-
apple chunks

1 scoop (2 tablespoons)
Pea Protein Powder
(page 18) or store-bought
protein powder

*This colorful, naturally sweet, and refreshing
smoothie is like a quick trip to the tropics after a
sweaty workout.*

1. Put the chia seeds and ½ cup of soy milk in a small
   bowl. Whisk to combine. Cover and refrigerate for
   about 10 minutes, until slightly thickened.

2. Put the banana, mango, pineapple, protein powder,
   and remaining 1 cup of soy milk in a high-speed
   blender. Blend on high speed until smooth.

3. Scrape the chia seed mixture into the blender and
   blend until smooth. Pour the shake into cold, tall
   glasses.

STORAGE: This shake can be frozen for up to 1 month and
thawed partially before serving.

SERVING TIP: For a delicious frozen treat, freeze the
smoothie mixture, then just scoop and eat it with a spoon.

PER SERVING (1 SMOOTHIE): Calories: 424; Protein: 23g; Total fat: 10g;
Carbohydrates: 67g; Fiber: 13g; Calcium: 386mg; Vitamin D: 89mg;
Vitamin B$_{12}$: 2mg; Iron: 5mg; Zinc: 3mg

MACROS: Protein 20%; Carbs 59%; Fat 21%

QUINOA BRITTLE

GLUTEN-FREE

QUENCH THE HUNGER

This crispy quinoa brittle is packed with nuts and seeds for extra protein. It makes an excellent afternoon snack, breakfast bowl topping, or crunchy add-in to your hot cereal. If you don't have sprouted quinoa, regular is fine for this recipe; just rinse it thoroughly in cool water and cook according to the package instructions.

SERVES 6

PREP TIME: 10 minutes

COOK TIME: 30 minutes

½ cup agave nectar

2 tablespoons coconut oil, melted

1 teaspoon vanilla extract

½ teaspoon sea salt

1 cup cooked or sprouted quinoa (see page 31 for sprouting instructions)

1 cup mixed nuts of choice, chopped

¼ cup pumpkin seeds

¼ cup sunflower seeds

2 tablespoons ground flaxseed

VARIATION: For a sweet treat, drizzle the cooled brittle with melted dark chocolate, and refrigerate to harden the chocolate.

1. Preheat the oven to 350°F. Line a baking sheet with parchment paper.

2. In a large bowl, whisk together the agave nectar, oil, vanilla, and salt until combined.

3. Fold in the quinoa, nuts, pumpkin seeds, sunflower seeds, and flaxseed. Stir until thoroughly combined.

4. Using a spatula, spread the quinoa mixture out in a thin layer on the prepared baking sheet.

5. Transfer the baking sheet to the oven and bake for 25 to 30 minutes, rotating halfway through, until the edges begin to turn golden. Check frequently so the brittle doesn't burn. Remove from the oven. Let cool, then break the brittle up into bite-size pieces.

STORAGE: Store in an airtight container in a cool, dry place for up to 3 weeks.

PER SERVING: Calories: 340; Protein: 8g; Total fat: 26g; Carbohydrates: 26g; Fiber: 6g; Calcium: 96mg; Vitamin D: 0mg; Vitamin B_{12}: 0mg; Iron: 2mg; Zinc: 2mg

MACROS: Protein 10%; Carbs 29%; Fat 61%

Vegan Sloppy Joes
page 84

5

ENERGIZING BOWLS, SALADS, AND SANDWICHES

As an athlete, you probably find yourself in many situations where it's better or just easier to bring your own food. Whether it's a quick bite after a lunchtime workout or a light evening meal before a training session, you need an arsenal of easy on-the-go meals to fuel your body.

This chapter will arm you with delicious, satisfying bowls, salads, and sandwiches to set you up for a great afternoon and energized evening. As a bonus, many of these recipes can be prepped ahead, so on-the-go meals are ready for the week. You'll also find some vegan twists on traditional flavors that are sure to delight you. The high protein will help you feel full and have plenty of energy to get through your day. Also, if you work out in the evening, you're setting yourself up for a power work-out and a great night's sleep.

SWEET POTATO, AVOCADO, AND LENTIL BOWLS

GLUTEN-FREE

HIGH-CARB

NUT-FREE

QUENCH THE HUNGER

RECOVERY BOOST

MAKES 4 BOWLS

PREP TIME: 20 minutes

COOK TIME: 30 to 35 minutes

1 large sweet potato, skin on, cut into ½-inch dice

1 head cauliflower, cut into large florets, stalk diced

2 garlic cloves

3 tablespoons avocado oil, divided

1 tablespoon garam masala (see tip)

Sea salt

Freshly ground black pepper

1½ cups dried green or red lentils

1 (1-inch) piece fresh ginger, grated

1 teaspoon whole-grain mustard

Sweet potatoes are a nutrition powerhouse—supporting immunity and vision. When they are combined with the protein and fiber in lentils, you have a nutrition-packed bowl. This Indian-inspired dish can be customized to your taste and is great for meal prepping, since it holds up very well in the refrigerator.

1. Preheat the oven to 375°F.

2. In a medium bowl, toss together the sweet potato, cauliflower, garlic, 1½ tablespoons of oil, the garam masala, pinch of salt, and pinch of pepper. Transfer to a large roasting pan.

3. Transfer the roasting pan to the oven and roast for 30 to 35 minutes, until the vegetables are golden brown and tender. Remove from the oven.

4. Meanwhile, put the lentils in a medium saucepan with enough cold water to cover by 1½ inches. Bring to a boil over medium-high heat.

5. Reduce the heat to low. Simmer for about 20 minutes, until the lentils are just tender. Remove from the heat. Drain and rinse under cool water.

6. Remove the garlic cloves from the roasting pan, place them in a large bowl, and mash them with a fork. Add the remaining 1½ tablespoons of oil, the ginger, mustard, and juice of 1 lime. Whisk to combine.

Juice of 2 limes, divided

2 medium carrots, grated

½ small head red cabbage, shredded

½ small bunch cilantro, chopped

1 medium ripe avocado, peeled, pitted, and sliced

7. Add the warm lentils to the bowl. Season with salt and pepper. Divide among 4 bowls (or 4 airtight containers if meal prepping).

8. To make the carrot slaw, in a medium bowl, combine the carrots, cabbage, cilantro, and juice of the remaining 1 lime. Season with salt and pepper as needed.

9. Top each serving equally with the carrot slaw, sweet potato and cauliflower mix, and avocado.

STORAGE: Store the bowls (minus the avocado) in the refrigerator for up to 5 days, or freeze for up to 3 months.

SWAP IT: Garam masala is an Indian spice blend that can contain more than 30 ingredients. It's a great pantry item that can add a little exciting flavor to your vegetables. If you don't have any on hand, you can mimic the basic flavor by combining 1 part cumin with ¼ part ground allspice.

PER SERVING (1 BOWL): Calories: 527; Protein: 22g; Total fat: 20g; Carbohydrates: 73g; Fiber: 17g; Calcium: 129mg; Vitamin D: 0mg; Vitamin B_{12}: 0mg; Iron: 7mg; Zinc: 3mg

MACROS: Protein 16%; Carbs 52%; Fat 32%

ROASTED VEGGIE AND BLACK BEAN SALSA QUINOA BOWLS

GLUTEN-FREE

NUT-FREE

QUENCH THE HUNGER

MAKES 4 BOWLS

PREP TIME: 15 minutes

COOK TIME: 20 minutes

FOR THE QUINOA

1 cup quinoa, rinsed

2 cups low-sodium vegetable stock

1 teaspoon sea salt, plus more as needed

¼ cup fresh cilantro leaves, chopped

¼ cup fresh basil leaves, chopped

Grated zest and juice of 1 lemon

Grain and bean bowls are vegan staples, but they can sometimes be uninspiring. This recipe changes everything! There's so much flavor packed into this delicious meal that is sure to satisfy your appetite and support your training. This is one of my favorite weeknight dinners.

TO MAKE THE QUINOA

1. In a medium saucepan, combine the quinoa, stock, and salt. Bring to a boil over medium-high heat. Stir and cover.

2. Reduce the heat to medium-low. Simmer for about 12 minutes, until the stock has been absorbed. Remove from the heat. Let sit, covered, for 5 minutes, then fluff the quinoa with a fork.

3. Fold the cilantro, basil, lemon zest, and lemon juice into the quinoa. Stir to combine. Taste and adjust the seasoning with salt as needed. Divide among 4 serving bowls.

FOR THE ROASTED VEGGIES

1 medium red
   onion, chopped

1 medium zucchini,
   chopped

1 pint cherry toma-
   toes, halved

1 tablespoon olive oil

1 teaspoon ground cumin

1 teaspoon smoked paprika

½ teaspoon sea salt, plus
   more as needed

Pinch cayenne pepper,
   plus more as needed
   (optional)

2 (15-ounce) cans
   black beans, drained
   and rinsed

TO MAKE THE ROASTED VEGGIES

4. Meanwhile, preheat the oven to 375°F. Line a baking sheet with parchment paper.

5. Put the onion, zucchini, and tomatoes on a baking sheet. Drizzle with the oil. Season with the cumin, paprika, salt, and cayenne (if using). Using your hands, toss the vegetables to combine. Spread out in an even layer.

6. Transfer the baking sheet to the oven and roast for 15 to 20 minutes, stirring once halfway through, until the vegetables are tender and beginning to brown. Remove from the oven.

7. Stir in the beans. Adjust the seasoning with more salt and cayenne as needed.

8. Top the quinoa with the roasted veggie and black bean salsa.

STORAGE: Refrigerate in a sealed container for up to 5 days, or freeze for up to 3 months.

VARIATION: Add optional toppings like avocado, scallions, vegan yogurt, or hot sauce.

PER SERVING (1 BOWL): Calories: 389; Protein: 20g; Total fat: 7g; Carbohydrates: 65g; Fiber: 16g; Calcium: 85mg; Vitamin D: 0mg; Vitamin B$_{12}$: 0mg; Iron: 5mg; Zinc: 3mg

MACROS: Protein 20%; Carbs 62%; Fat 18%

SPROUTED GRAIN AND CURRIED CAULIFLOWER BOWLS

HIGH-CARB

NUT-FREE

QUENCH THE HUNGER

If you've never cooked with rye before, you're in for a treat. Rye is my favorite grain because of its distinct flavor, but any type of sprouted grain (see page 31 for instructions) will work.

MAKES 4 BOWLS

PREP TIME: 10 minutes

COOK TIME: 30 minutes

1 large head cauliflower, divided into florets

1 tablespoon olive oil, plus ¼ cup

1 teaspoon sea salt

1 teaspoon curry powder

½ teaspoon smoked paprika

4 cups sprouted rye berries or sprouted grain of choice

1 (15-ounce) can chickpeas, drained and rinsed

½ cup pumpkin seeds

¼ cup sliced scallions, green and white parts

2 teaspoons Pea Protein Powder (page 18), or store-bought

Grated zest and juice of 1 large lemon

½ teaspoon freshly ground black pepper

1. Preheat the oven to 400°F. Line a baking sheet with parchment paper.

2. In a bowl, toss together the cauliflower, 1 tablespoon of oil, the salt, curry powder, and paprika.

3. Spread the cauliflower out in a single layer on the prepared baking sheet.

4. Transfer the baking sheet to the oven and roast for about 30 minutes, until the cauliflower is tender and golden. Remove from the oven.

5. In a large skillet, warm the rye berries and chickpeas slightly, or microwave for about 1 minute. Remove from the heat.

6. In a large bowl, toss together the rye berries, chickpeas, cauliflower, pumpkin seeds, scallions, protein powder, remaining ¼ cup of olive oil, the lemon zest, lemon juice, and pepper. Adjust the seasoning with more salt and pepper as needed.

STORAGE: Store in the refrigerator for up to 5 days, or freeze for up to 2 months.

PER SERVING (1 BOWL): Calories: 652; Protein: 28g; Total fat: 28g; Carbohydrates: 47g; Fiber: 12g; Calcium: 143mg; Vitamin D: 0mg; Vitamin B_{12}: 0mg; Iron: 8mg; Zinc: 5mg

MACROS: Protein 15%; Carbs 47%; Fat 38%

CHICKPEA, ARUGULA, AND VEGAN CHEESE SALAD

GLUTEN-FREE

LOW-CARB

SERVES 2

PREP TIME: 20 minutes

1 (15-ounce) can chickpeas, drained and rinsed

1 medium red bell pepper, cored and diced

1 English cucumber, diced

1 pint cherry tomatoes, halved

1 small red onion, chopped

¼ cup pitted Kalamata olives, quartered

½ cup crumbled Vegan Soft Cheese (page 24) or store-bought dairy-free soft cheese

2 tablespoons coarsely chopped fresh dill

½ cup Green Goddess Dressing (page 28)

Sea salt

Freshly ground black pepper

2 cups arugula

This classic Greek-style salad is a snap to make and is loaded with crunchy vegetables. It's also as versatile as you want it to be. Feel free to mix up the protein, vegetables, herbs, and greens to your taste.

1. In a large bowl, combine the chickpeas, bell pepper, cucumber, tomatoes, onion, olives, cheese, and dill.

2. Add the dressing and toss well to combine. Adjust the seasoning with salt and pepper.

3. Divide the arugula among 2 serving bowls.

4. Top each bowl with the chickpea mixture.

STORAGE: The chickpea mixture can be refrigerated in a sealed container for up to 1 week. Just pull it out and toss it with the greens when you are ready to eat.

PER SERVING: Calories: 608; Protein: 22g; Total fat: 34g; Carbohydrates: 58g; Fiber: 14g; Calcium: 216mg; Vitamin D: 2mg; Vitamin B$_{12}$: 0mg; Iron: 6mg; Zinc: 4mg

MACROS: Protein 14%; Carbs 36%; Fat 50%

TOFU SATAY AND QUINOA BOWLS

HIGH-CARB

QUENCH THE HUNGER

RECOVERY BOOST

These zingy, Asian-inspired bowls are excellent for meal prepping and packing for weekday lunches. For a variation, cook the marinated tofu on the grill.

MAKES 4 BOWLS

PREP TIME: 20 minutes, plus 2 hours to marinate

COOK TIME: 20 minutes

FOR THE TOFU AND QUINOA

1 tablespoon avocado oil

1 tablespoon soy sauce

1 tablespoon pure maple syrup

1 teaspoon Sriracha sauce

½ teaspoon ground turmeric

1 tablespoon grated fresh ginger

1 garlic clove, minced

1 (14-ounce) package extra-firm tofu, drained, pressed, and cut into 1-inch dice

2 tablespoons cornstarch

2½ cups water or vegetable stock

1 cup quinoa, rinsed

Sea salt

TO MAKE THE TOFU AND QUINOA

1. In a large bowl, combine the oil, soy sauce, maple syrup, Sriracha, turmeric, ginger, and garlic.

2. Add the tofu and toss well to coat thoroughly. Cover and set aside for at least 2 hours or overnight.

3. Preheat the oven to 400°F. Line a baking sheet with parchment paper.

4. Drain the tofu. Transfer to a bowl. Toss with the cornstarch to coat.

5. Spread the tofu out in an even layer on the prepared baking sheet.

6. Transfer the baking sheet to the oven and bake for about 20 minutes, until the tofu is golden brown and crispy. Remove from the oven.

7. Meanwhile, in a medium saucepan, combine the water and quinoa. Season with salt. Bring to a boil over medium-high heat.

8. Reduce the heat to medium-low. Cover the saucepan and simmer for about 12 minutes, until the liquid has been absorbed. Remove from the heat. Divide among 4 serving bowls.

FOR THE SATAY SAUCE

¼ cup peanut butter

3 tablespoons hot water

1 tablespoon soy sauce

1 tablespoon freshly
   squeezed lime juice

1 teaspoon pure
   maple syrup

1 teaspoon Sriracha sauce

1 teaspoon rice vinegar

TO MAKE THE SATAY SAUCE

9. While the quinoa is cooking, in a small bowl, whisk together the peanut butter, water, soy sauce, lime juice, maple syrup, Sriracha, and vinegar until smooth and creamy.

10. Top the quinoa with the tofu, and drizzle with the satay sauce.

11. Garnish with your toppings of choice, such as cucumber slices, pickled red onion, coarsely chopped cilantro or peanuts, or toasted sesame seeds.

STORAGE: The marinated tofu and satay sauce will keep for 3 days in the refrigerator; the satay sauce can be frozen for up to 6 months.

SWAP IT: The satay sauce here is super quick, but if you want to save time or ingredients, pick up a store-bought organic satay sauce.

PER SERVING (1 BOWL): Calories: 415; Protein: 20g; Total fat: 20g; Carbohydrates: 42g; Fiber: 4g; Calcium: 213mg; Vitamin D: 0mg; Vitamin B$_{12}$: 0mg; Iron: 4mg; Zinc: 3mg

MACROS: Protein 18%; Carbs 40%; Fat 42%

SPROUTED LENTIL, BELL PEPPER, AND CUCUMBER POWER SALAD

SERVES 3

PREP TIME: 20 minutes

¼ cup extra-virgin olive oil

¼ cup apple cider vinegar

1 tablespoon pure
maple syrup

1 tablespoon
stone-ground mustard

2 small garlic
cloves, minced

2 teaspoons sea salt, plus
more as needed

1 teaspoon freshly ground
black pepper, plus more
as needed

5 cups sprouted lentils (see
page 31)

1 medium English cucum-
ber, diced

1 large red onion, diced

1 large red bell pepper,
cored and diced

3 celery stalks, thinly sliced

1 cup dried tart cherries

1 cup sliced almonds

2 cups baby arugula

This lentil salad is loaded with nutrient-dense vegetables and protein-packed lentils. It makes enough for a family dinner or for several make-ahead meals. I love this with toasted slices of crusty wheat bread.

1. In a large bowl, whisk together the oil, vinegar, maple syrup, mustard, garlic, salt, and black pepper until well combined.

2. Add the lentils, cucumber, onion, bell pepper, and celery. Toss to combine. Adjust the seasoning with salt and pepper as needed.

3. Add the dried cherries and almonds.

4. Serve the salad immediately over a bed of arugula.

STORAGE: The lentils can be prepared and refrigerated in an airtight container for up to 1 week.

MAKE AHEAD: Toss the lentils with the dried cherries and sliced almonds ahead of time, and serve over the arugula when ready to eat.

PER SERVING: Calories: 673; Protein: 20g; Total fat: 35g; Carbohydrates: 83g; Fiber: 11g; Calcium: 208mg; Vitamin D: 0mg; Vitamin B12: 0mg; Iron: 5mg; Zinc: 3mg

MACROS: Protein 9%; Carbs 46%; Fat 45%

BLACKENED TEMPEH SANDWICHES

HIGH-CARB

NUT-FREE

QUENCH THE HUNGER

MAKES 2 SANDWICHES

PREP TIME: 15 minutes

COOK TIME: 10 to 15 minutes

3 tablespoons Vegan
    Mayonnaise (page 25)
    or store-bought

1 tablespoon
    whole-grain mustard

2 teaspoons hot sauce, or
    to taste

1 garlic clove, minced

Pinch cayenne pepper

2 tablespoons bal-
    samic vinegar

2 tablespoons Cajun or
    blackening seasoning

2 tablespoons coconut oil

1 (8-ounce) package
    tempeh, cut into
    4 even slices

4 sprouted wheat bread
    slices, lightly toasted

½ cup arugula

STORAGE: Store in the
refrigerator for up to
5 days, or freeze for
1 month.

*These sandwiches are packed with spicy flavor!
Made with blackened tempeh, greens, and creamy
vegan remoulade sauce, they cook in minutes and
are perfect for lunch or dinner.*

1. To make the sauce, in a small bowl, combine
   the mayonnaise, mustard, hot sauce, garlic, and
   cayenne.

2. In a small bowl, whisk together the vinegar and
   Cajun seasoning.

3. In a large skillet, melt the oil over medium heat
   until it begins to shimmer.

4. Working in batches if needed, add the tempeh and
   cook for about 2 minutes, until lightly golden.

5. Flip the tempeh and cook for 2 minutes or
   until golden.

6. Spoon the balsamic vinegar mixture over the
   tempeh, then flip so the seasoned side faces
   down. Cook for 1 to 2 minutes, until the seasoning
   blackens and becomes crispy. Repeat on the other
   side. Remove from the heat. Transfer to a plate and
   keep warm.

7. Spread the Cajun sauce onto the bread.

8. Top 2 slices of bread with a handful of arugula,
   followed by the blackened tempeh. Top with the
   remaining 2 slices of bread. Enjoy immediately.

PER SERVING (1 SANDWICH): Calories: 593; Protein: 31g; Total fat: 36g;
Carbohydrates: 43g; Fiber: 5g; Calcium: 261mg; Vitamin D: 0mg;
Vitamin B$_{12}$: 0mg; Iron: 5mg; Zinc: 3mg

MACROS: Protein 19%; Carbs 29%; Fat 52%

GREEK POWER SALAD

GLUTEN-FREE

QUENCH THE HUNGER

SERVES 4

PREP TIME: 15 minutes

COOK TIME: 15 minutes

2 cups water

1 cup quinoa, rinsed

4 cups chopped
romaine hearts

2 cups canned butter
beans or any kind
of beans

1 small English cucum-
ber, diced

1 cup halved cherry
tomatoes

½ cup pitted and halved
Kalamata olives

½ cup toasted almonds

½ cup Vegan Caesar
Dressing (page 29), or
store-bought

½ cup Vegan Soft
Cheese (page 24), or
store-bought

¼ cup fresh parsley
leaves, chopped

I love a traditional Greek salad, and for this one, I've added some power ingredients to increase the protein and fiber. In addition to being delicious, it's filling and satisfying as an entrée. The butter beans in this recipe are known as gigantes in Greece because of their size.

1. In a small saucepan, combine the water and quinoa. Bring to a boil over medium-high heat.

2. Reduce the heat to low. Cover the saucepan and simmer for 15 minutes. Remove from the heat. Let sit, covered, for 5 minutes. Using a fine-mesh strainer, drain the quinoa. Rinse under cold water to stop the cooking process.

3. In a large bowl, toss together the quinoa, romaine, beans, cucumber, tomatoes, olives, almonds, and dressing. Divide among 4 serving bowls.

4. Sprinkle with the cheese and parsley.

STORAGE: This is an excellent make-ahead salad; simply combine all the vegetables except the romaine, transfer the mixture to an airtight container, and refrigerate for up to 1 week. When ready to serve, toss with the romaine and dressing, and garnish with the cheese and parsley.

SERVING TIP: The bean salad on its own makes a great side dish or bowl component.

PER SERVING: Calories: 565; Protein: 22g; Total fat: 27g; Carbohydrates: 63g; Fiber: 17g; Calcium: 213mg; Vitamin D: 2mg; Vitamin B$_{12}$: 0mg; Iron: 7mg; Zinc: 3mg

MACROS: Protein 15%; Carbs 44%; Fat 41%

THAI PEANUT NOODLE SALAD

SERVES 3

PREP TIME: 30 minutes

COOK TIME: 15 minutes

6 ounces high-protein
   pasta noodles

¼ cup creamy natural
   peanut butter

Juice of 1 orange

Juice of 1 lime

3 thin slices fresh ginger

1 large garlic clove

3 tablespoons agave nectar

3 tablespoons toasted
   sesame oil

2 tablespoons soy sauce

½ teaspoon cayenne
   pepper

½ teaspoon sea salt, plus
   more as needed

1 small head cabbage,
   cored and thinly sliced

2 medium carrots, grated

1 red bell pepper, cored
   and thinly sliced

3 scallions, green and
   white parts, thinly sliced

½ bunch fresh cilantro
   leaves, coarsely chopped

This crave-worthy, make-ahead salad is perfect for midweek meals and portable lunches. You might be tempted to eat the delectable peanut butter–citrus sauce with a spoon by itself! Top with grilled tofu or Basic Seitan (page 20) for extra protein.

1. Bring a medium pot of water to a boil over high heat. Cook the noodles according to the package instructions. Drain and run under cold water to stop the cooking process.

2. Meanwhile, to make the peanut sauce, put the peanut butter, orange juice, lime juice, ginger, garlic, agave nectar, sesame oil, soy sauce, cayenne, and salt in a high-speed blender. Blend until smooth.

3. Put the cabbage, carrots, bell pepper, scallions, and cilantro in a large mixing bowl. Toss to combine.

4. Add the noodles to the bowl and toss again.

5. Add the peanut sauce and toss well to coat. Adjust the seasoning with salt as needed. Divide among 4 serving bowls.

STORAGE: Refrigerate in a sealed container for up to 5 days; I don't suggest freezing.

PER SERVING: Calories: 584; Protein: 22g; Total fat: 27g; Carbohydrates: 81g; Fiber: 13g; Calcium: 189mg; Vitamin D: 0mg; Vitamin B$_{12}$: 0mg; Iron: 4mg; Zinc: 1mg

MACROS: Protein 14%; Carbs 48%; Fat 38%

BBQ JACKFRUIT SANDWICHES

NUT-FREE

QUENCH THE HUNGER

MAKES 6 SANDWICHES

PREP TIME: 15 minutes
COOK TIME: 1 hour
10 minutes

2 tablespoons olive oil

1 medium yellow
onion, sliced

3 garlic cloves, minced

3 cups canned jackfruit,
drained and patted dry

2 cups cooked lentils

2 teaspoons sea salt

1 tablespoon Mediter-
ranean Spice Blend
(page 30)

1 teaspoon vegan Worces-
tershire sauce

½ teaspoon cay-
enne pepper

2 cups low-sodium vegeta-
ble stock

½ cup barbecue sauce

6 sprouted wheat sand-
wich buns

Dairy-free coleslaw, for
serving (optional; see tip)

Jackfruit is a vegan's dream food, with a texture that both simulates meat and absorbs flavors easily. This recipe, which is a vegan version of pulled pork, can fool a carnivore! The addition of cooked lentils sneaks in some extra protein with-out taking away any of the flavor.

1. Preheat the oven to 375°F. Line a baking sheet with parchment paper.

2. In a Dutch oven, heat the oil over medium heat. Add the onion and garlic. Cook for about 4 minutes, until softened and translucent. Add the jackfruit, lentils, salt, spice blend, Worcestershire sauce, and cayenne. Stir to coat evenly. Add the stock and bring to a simmer.

3. Reduce the heat to low. Cover the Dutch oven and simmer for about 10 minutes, until the liquid has mostly reduced and the flavors have combined. Remove from the heat.

4. Spread the jackfruit out on the prepared baking sheet.

5. Transfer the baking sheet to the oven and bake for 30 to 35 minutes, until the jackfruit has dried and becomes a deeper golden brown. Remove from the oven, leaving the oven on.

6. Pour the barbecue sauce over the jackfruit. Toss to combine, then return the baking sheet to the oven for 15 minutes. Remove from the oven.

7. Serve the barbecue jackfruit warm on the buns with dairy-free coleslaw (if using).

STORAGE: The jackfruit mixture can be refrigerated in an airtight container for up to 1 week or frozen for up to 6 months.

INGREDIENT TIP: Coleslaw mix tossed with cider vinegar, a bit of sugar, salt, and a drizzle of olive oil makes a pleasing topping for these sandwiches. Or try using the Vegan Mayonnaise on page 25.

PER SERVING (2 SANDWICHES): Calories: 726; Protein: 24g; Total fat: 14g; Carbohydrates: 132g; Fiber: 16g; Calcium: 244mg; Vitamin D: 0mg; Vitamin B$_{12}$: 0mg; Iron: 8mg; Zinc: 2mg

MACROS: Protein 13%; Carbs 70%; Fat 17%

VEGAN SLOPPY JOES

HIGH-CARB

NUT-FREE

QUENCH THE HUNGER

MAKES 4 SANDWICHES

PREP TIME: 15 minutes

COOK TIME: 35 to 40 minutes

2 cups low-sodium vegetable stock

1½ cups dried green lentils, well rinsed

2 tablespoons olive oil

1 small yellow onion, minced

1 small red bell pepper, cored and diced

2 garlic cloves, minced

Sea salt

Freshly ground black pepper

1 (15-ounce) can tomato sauce (see tip)

2 tablespoons coconut sugar (see tip), plus more as needed

2 tablespoons vegan Worcestershire sauce, plus more as needed

2 teaspoons chili powder, plus more as needed

This savory, sweet, and spicy sandwich is a fabulous plant-forward choice for a crowd—everyone loves sloppy joes! This version made with lentils, which replace traditional ground beef, is as good as the original and full of vegetables and protein. Add some corn kernels to the mixture for an additional pop of sweetness.

1. In a large saucepan, combine the stock and lentils. Bring to a boil over medium-high heat.

2. Reduce the heat to low. Simmer for 18 to 20 minutes, until the lentils are just tender. Remove from the heat. Drain and rinse under cold water to stop the cooking process.

3. After the lentils have cooked for 15 minutes, heat the oil in a large skillet over medium heat.

4. When the oil begins to shimmer, add the onion, bell pepper, and garlic. Season with a bit of salt and pepper. Stir to combine. Sauté for 5 minutes, stirring frequently, or until the onion and bell pepper are tender and golden brown.

5. Add the tomato sauce, sugar, Worcestershire sauce, chili powder, cumin, and paprika. Stir to combine.

6. Once the lentils have cooked, add them to the skillet and stir to combine.

7. Reduce the heat to low. Cook for 5 to 10 minutes, stirring occasionally, until the mixture thickens to the texture you like. Taste and adjust the flavor as needed, adding more chili powder, sugar, or Worcestershire to balance flavors. Remove from the heat.

1 teaspoon ground cumin

Pinch smoked paprika

**Sprouted wheat ham-
burger buns or buns of
choice, toasted**

8. Spoon the hot mixture onto the buns and top with your favorite toppings. I recommend shredded cabbage and vegan cheese.

STORAGE: Refrigerate in an airtight container for up to 5 days, or freeze for 1 month.

INGREDIENT TIP: Canned tomato sauces can be high in sodium. Most athletes don't need to worry too much about sodium, since it helps replace sweat losses. However, it's still a good idea to check the nutrition label for sodium content. Lower sodium options are available when needed.

VARIATION: I like to use coconut sugar, because it has a delicious caramel flavor and a lower glycemic index than regular sugar. If you don't have it, use light brown sugar.

PER SERVING (1 SANDWICH): Calories: 508; Protein: 24g; Total fat: 10g; Carbohydrates: 83g; Fiber: 12g; Calcium: 141mg; Vitamin D: 0mg; Vitamin B$_{12}$: 0mg; Iron: 9mg; Zinc: 3mg

MACROS: Protein 18%; Carbs 64%; Fat 18%

GRAB 'N' GO BEAN BURRITOS

HIGH-CARB

NUT-FREE

QUENCH THE HUNGER

RECOVERY BOOST

MAKES 10 BURRITOS

PREP TIME: 30 minutes

COOK TIME: 30 minutes

1 medium zucchini, diced

1 medium red bell pepper,
cored and diced

1 medium red onion, diced

8 ounces cremini (or
any variety) mush-
rooms, sliced

2 tablespoons olive oil

1½ teaspoons sea
salt, divided

½ teaspoon ground cumin

½ teaspoon dried oregano

1½ cups brown rice or
grain of choice

½ tablespoon chili powder

3 cups water

10 (12-inch) whole-wheat or
gluten-free tortillas

2 (15-ounce) cans
black beans, drained
and rinsed

2½ cups shredded vegan
pepper Jack cheese

Leaves from 1 bunch fresh
cilantro

These roasted vegetable burritos are easy and inexpensive and might become a meal prep staple. Once assembled, they can be wrapped individually and frozen. Then, pop one in the oven or microwave for a grab 'n' go breakfast or lunch.

1. Preheat the oven to 400°F. Line a baking sheet with parchment paper.

2. In a large bowl, combine the zucchini, bell pepper, onion, mushrooms, oil, ½ teaspoon of salt, the cumin, and oregano. Toss until the vegetables are thoroughly coated.

3. Spread the vegetables out on the prepared baking sheet.

4. Transfer the baking sheet to the oven and roast, stirring occasionally to ensure even browning, for 30 minutes. Remove from the oven.

5. Meanwhile, in a medium saucepan, combine the rice, remaining 1 teaspoon of salt, the chili powder, and water. Cover and bring to a boil over high heat.

6. Reduce the heat to low. Simmer for 20 minutes or until the liquid has been absorbed and the rice is tender. Remove from the heat. Keep covered.

7. To make the burritos, lay the tortillas on a large plate, cover with a damp paper towel, and microwave for 30 seconds to soften.

8. Uncover the rice and fluff with a fork. Place about ¼ cup of rice on each tortilla.

9. Top each tortilla with ¼ cup of beans, ¼ cup of roasted vegetables, and ¼ cup of cheese.

10. Sprinkle with the cilantro. Fold up the sides of the tortillas, roll the burritos tightly lengthwise, and enjoy while hot.

STORAGE: Wrap tightly in plastic wrap and refrigerate for up to 5 days, or freeze for up to 6 months.

VARIATION: Your favorite salsa and vegan yogurt are delicious additions.

PER SERVING (2 BURRITOS): Calories: 820; Protein: 30g; Total fat: 24g; Carbohydrates: 124g; Fiber: 22g, Calcium: 608mg; Vitamin D: 4mg; Vitamin B_{12}: 0mg; Iron: 6mg; Zinc: 6mg

MACROS: Protein 14%; Carbs 61%; Fat 25%

TEMPEH, AVOCADO, AND SUN-DRIED TOMATO HUMMUS WRAPS

SERVES 2

PREP TIME: 5 minutes

COOK TIME: 10 minutes

2 teaspoons olive oil

1 (8-ounce) package
   tempeh, sliced

2 tablespoons pure maple
   syrup, plus 2 teaspoons

2 tablespoons tamari or
   soy sauce

¼ teaspoon
   smoked paprika

1 teaspoon sea salt,
   plus pinch

½ teaspoon freshly ground
   black pepper

½ cup hummus

¼ cup sun-dried tomatoes
   in olive oil, chopped

2 tablespoons Vegan
   Mayonnaise (page 25) or
   store-bought

1 tablespoon Sriracha
   sauce

This wrap is simple to prepare and boasts a surprising amount of flavor. Tempeh is a meaty, textured, plant-based protein that absorbs flavor beautifully. Make this wrap to take on the go, and you'll be the envy of anyone you find yourself eating with.

1. In a medium skillet, heat the oil over medium heat until it begins to shimmer.

2. Add the tempeh and cook for about 2 minutes per side, until golden.

3. Meanwhile, in a small bowl, whisk together 2 tablespoons of maple syrup, the tamari, paprika, 1 teaspoon of salt, and pepper.

4. Reduce the heat to low. Add the maple syrup mixture to the skillet, turning the tempeh over to coat both sides. Cook for another 2 minutes per side, until golden brown and caramelized. Remove from the heat.

5. While the tempeh is cooking, in a small bowl, whisk together the hummus, sun-dried tomatoes, vegan mayonnaise, and Sriracha.

6. Warm the tortillas.

7. Using a fork, smash the avocado onto the tortillas. Sprinkle with the remaining pinch of salt.

8. Drizzle 1 tablespoon of the maple syrup mixture over the avocado, then top with a layer of the hummus mixture.

**2 (12-inch) wraps or
tortillas**

**½ ripe avocado, pitted,
peeled, and sliced**

**1 cup watercress or greens
of choice**

9. Top with the tempeh and watercress. Roll up the
    wraps and slice in half diagonally.

STORAGE: I recommend eating these right away; the
hummus mixture can be made ahead and refrigerated in a
sealed container for 1 week.

VARIATION: Serve this delicious sautéed tempeh in a taco,
on toasted bread, or as a salad or bowl component.

PER SERVING (1 WRAP): Calories: 659; Protein: 31g; Total fat: 38g;
Carbohydrates: 55g; Fiber: 8g; Calcium: 255mg; Vitamin D: 0mg;
Vitamin B$_{12}$: 0mg; Iron: 6mg; Zinc: 3mg

MACROS: Protein 17%; Carbs 33%; Fat 50%

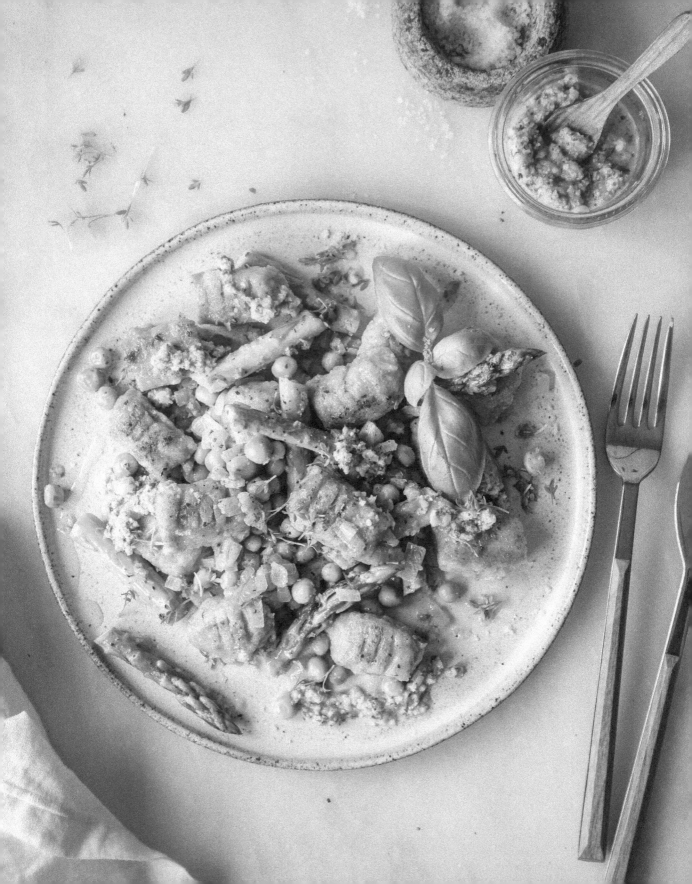

6

PROTEIN-PACKED DINNERS

If you're bored with your dinner routine, then you've come to the right place. This mouthwatering collection will take you around the world, exposing you to new techniques and flavors. But don't be intimidated; these approachable recipes are doable and will help you learn how to build flavor in dishes (which sounds more complicated than it is). Many recipes offer options to customize the ingredients to meet your specific energy needs. Don't shy away from adding more carbohydrates when you really need them! Remember to listen to your body, and provide what it needs to thrive.

**Gnocchi with Chickpeas
and Basil-Walnut Pesto**
page 110

RED LENTIL DAL

GLUTEN-FREE

HIGH-CARB

NUT-FREE

QUENCH THE HUNGER

RECOVERY BOOST

SERVES 2

PREP TIME: 10 minutes

COOK TIME: 45 minutes

2 tablespoons olive oil

1 medium yellow onion,
    finely diced

1 teaspoon sea salt, plus
    more as needed

1 medium sweet potato,
    peeled and finely diced

1 (3-inch) piece fresh
    ginger, grated

2 garlic cloves, minced

1 Thai chile, seeded and
    minced (optional)

1 cup dried red lentils

2 teaspoons ground cumin

2 teaspoons ground
    turmeric

1 (15-ounce) can
    fire-roasted diced
    tomatoes

1 quart low-sodium
    vegetable stock

This spiced red lentil stew studded with sweet potato and tomatoes is packed with protein, fiber, and antioxidants. Dal is so simple, because it all but cooks itself, and it tastes better the longer it is stored, always a bonus in my book. This dal is excellent with sautéed or grilled Basic Seitan (page 20). I love it with steamed brown rice or topped with cilantro and unsweetened toasted coconut shavings.

1. In a large, heavy-bottomed stockpot or Dutch oven, heat the oil over medium-low heat until it begins to shimmer.

2. Add the onion and salt. Sauté for about 2 minutes, until softened.

3. Add the sweet potato and sauté for 5 minutes.

4. Add the ginger and garlic. Stir.

5. Reduce the heat to low. Add the chile (if using), lentils, cumin, and turmeric. Stir until thoroughly combined.

6. Add the tomatoes with their juices and the stock.

7. Increase the heat to medium-high. Bring to a boil.

8. Reduce the heat to medium-low. Simmer for about 20 minutes, stirring occasionally, until the lentils and sweet potato are tender. Adjust the seasoning with salt as needed. Continue to simmer for 10 minutes or until the mixture has reduced and thickened.

9. Whisk the lentils and sweet potato, and mash the mixture lightly against the side of the pot to create a thick stew. Remove from the heat. Divide among warm serving bowls, and serve immediately.

STORAGE: Refrigerate in an airtight container for up to 1 week, or freeze for up to 6 months.

VARIATION: Use a can of light coconut milk in place of half of the vegetable stock for an extra-rich and hearty dal, especially nice in winter.

PER SERVING: Calories: 598; Protein: 28g; Total fat: 16g; Carbohydrates: 90g; Fiber: 18g; Calcium: 180mg; Vitamin D: 0mg; Vitamin B12: 0mg; Iron: 12mg; Zinc: 4mg

MACROS: Protein 15%; Carbs 60%; Fat 25%

BUTTERNUT SQUASH, LENTIL, AND WHITE BEAN CHILI

GLUTEN-FREE

HIGH-CARB

NUT-FREE

QUENCH THE HUNGER

SERVES 4

PREP TIME: 15 minutes

COOK TIME: 40 to 45 minutes

2 tablespoons olive oil

1 medium onion, diced

1 large yellow bell pepper, cored and diced

4 garlic cloves, minced

2 cups dried lentils, rinsed

1 tablespoon chili powder, plus more as needed

2 teaspoons ground cumin

2 teaspoons dried oregano

Sea salt

Freshly ground black pepper

7 cups low-sodium vegetable stock

1 (32-ounce) can diced fire-roasted tomatoes

1 bay leaf

You won't miss the meat in this wholesome, filling chili, which is easy to make with simple pantry ingredients. This is a speedy and warming week-night meal that's ideal for meal prepping, too. I usually make a double batch and freeze some indi-vidual portions for easy-to-reheat lunches.

1. In a large, heavy-bottomed pot or Dutch oven, heat the oil over medium heat.

2. Add the onion and bell pepper. Sauté for 5 to 6 minutes, until the vegetables begin to soften.

3. Stir in the garlic and cook for 30 seconds or until aromas are released.

4. Add the lentils, chili powder, cumin, and oregano. Season with salt and pepper. Cook, stirring con-stantly, for about 1 minute.

5. Add the stock, tomatoes with their juices, and bay leaf. Bring to a boil.

6. Reduce the heat to low. Partially cover the pan and simmer for 10 to 15 minutes, until the lentils are just tender.

7. Add the squash and simmer for about 10 minutes, until the squash is just tender.

1 (2-pound) butternut squash, peeled, seeded, and diced (or frozen and thawed butternut squash)

1 (15-ounce) can white beans, drained and rinsed

8. Stir in the beans and cook for 2 to 3 minutes, until heated through. Remove from the heat. Season with salt and pepper. Discard the bay leaf. Serve the chili with your favorite toppings.

STORAGE: Refrigerate in an airtight container for up to 5 days, or freeze for up to 6 months.

SERVING TIP: Topping options might include sliced scallions, chopped red onion, pickled jalapeños, shredded plant-based cheese, and tortilla strips.

PER SERVING: Calories: 643; Protein: 35g; Total fat: 9g; Carbohydrates: 114g; Fiber: 24g; Calcium: 292mg; Vitamin D: 0mg; Vitamin B_{12}: 0mg; Iron: 13mg; Zinc: 5mg

MACROS: Protein 18%; Carbs 69%; Fat 13%

PUMPKIN, CASHEW, AND QUINOA CURRY

GLUTEN-FREE

LOW-CARB

QUENCH THE HUNGER

SERVES 4

PREP TIME: 15 minutes

COOK TIME: 25 minutes

2 cups dried green lentils

2 tablespoons avocado
oil, divided

4½ cups fresh or frozen
diced pumpkin or any
variety of winter squash

1 teaspoon curry powder
or paste

2 small red onions, halved
and cut into thick
half-moons

2 garlic cloves, minced

1 (1-inch) piece fresh
ginger, grated

1 Thai chile, seeded and
minced, or 1 teaspoon red
pepper flakes (optional)

¾ cup unsalted
roasted cashews

1½ cups unsweetened
coconut milk

*This easy, creamy curry tastes a lot more com-
plicated than it really is to make. It'll feel like a
warm hug to your belly, especially after a hard
day of training. If you don't have time to make the
Quinoa Pilaf, serve this over plain cooked quinoa
or brown rice.*

1. Combine the lentils and 4 cups of water in a
    medium pot over high heat. Bring to a boil, then
    reduce the heat to low, cover, and cook for about
    20 minutes until tender but not mushy. Set aside.

2. Meanwhile, in a large saucepan, heat 1 tablespoon
    of oil over medium heat. Add the pumpkin and
    cook, stirring occasionally, for 8 to 10 minutes, until
    golden. Using a slotted spoon, transfer the cooked
    pumpkin to a plate.

3. Add the remaining 1 tablespoon of oil to the same
    saucepan.

4. Add the curry powder and toast, stirring constantly,
    for about 30 seconds.

5. Add the onions, garlic, and ginger. Sauté for about
    4 minutes, until the onions are golden.

6. Add the chile (if using) and cashews. Cook, stirring
    constantly, for 1 minute.

7. Add the coconut milk and coconut cream.

8. Increase the heat to medium-high. Simmer for
    about 2 minutes, until the mixture has thickened.

1 cup unsweetened
   coconut cream (see tip)
½ small bunch fresh
   cilantro, coarsely
   chopped, plus more
   for garnish
Juice of 1 lime (optional)
1 recipe Quinoa Pilaf
   (page 32)
Lime wedges, for garnish
   (optional)

9. Return the pumpkin to the saucepan, and reduce the heat to medium-low. Simmer for about 5 minutes, until the pumpkin is tender. Remove from the heat and add the cooked lentils.

10. Stir in the cilantro and lime juice (if using).

11. Spoon the curry over the warm quinoa pilaf.

12. Garnish with additional cilantro sprigs and lime wedges (if using).

STORAGE: Refrigerate in an airtight container for up to 1 week, or freeze for up to 1 month.

COOKING TIP: Don't confuse coconut cream with the sweet cream of coconut used for baking or cocktails. Coconut cream is a richer version of coconut milk that is made from pressed coconut. If you can't find it, use more coconut milk.

PER SERVING: Calories: 683; Protein: 22g; Total fat: 43g; Carbohydrates: 52g; Fiber: 12g; Calcium: 191mg; Vitamin D: 0mg; Vitamin B_{12}: 0mg; Iron: 3mg; Zinc: 3mg

MACROS: Protein 13%; Carbs 30%; Fat 57%

SWEET POTATO AND COCONUT BROWN RICE SUSHI ROLLS

MAKES 12 ROLLS

PREP TIME: 10 minutes

COOK TIME: 25 minutes

4 tablespoons tamari

4 tablespoons pure maple syrup

4 tablespoons sunflower seeds, coarsely chopped

4 large sweet potatoes, peeled and cut lengthwise into ½-inch-thick strips

4 cups brown rice

4 cups light unsweetened coconut milk

4 cups water

3 tablespoons rice vinegar

1 teaspoon sea salt

12 nori sheets

2 large English cucumbers, cut lengthwise into strips

2 teaspoons toasted sesame seeds

Sushi is easy and fun to make. You don't even need any special equipment. I love to add seeds to vegetable sushi for extra protein and a delicious crunch. Pumpkin seeds and crushed walnuts are delicious, but experiment with your own favorites.

1. Preheat the oven to 375°F. Line a baking sheet with parchment paper.

2. In a medium bowl, stir together the tamari and maple syrup.

3. Spread the sunflower seeds out on a plate.

4. Dip the sweet potatoes in the tamari mixture to coat, then press them into the sunflower seeds to coat on both sides.

5. Lay the sweet potatoes on the prepared baking sheet in a single layer.

6. Transfer the baking sheet to the oven. Bake for about 25 minutes, turning the baking sheet halfway through, until the sweet potatoes are tender and golden.

7. Meanwhile, in a small saucepan, combine the rice, coconut milk, water, vinegar, and salt. Bring to a simmer over high heat.

8. Reduce the heat to low. Cover the saucepan and simmer for about 20 minutes, until the liquid has been absorbed and the rice is tender. Remove from the heat. Let sit for 5 minutes, then spread the rice out on a plate; let it cool to room temperature.

9. Place a sheet of parchment paper (or a sushi mat, if you have one) on a clean work surface. Dampen your fingers lightly with water. Place a sheet of nori on the paper.

10. Using your fingers, cover the nori with a thin layer of rice.

11. Arrange the sweet potatoes evenly in a single row along the width of the nori sheet, about 1 inch from the edge.

12. Place a few cucumber strips next to the sweet potatoes.

13. Using the parchment paper, lift the end of the nori sheet and tightly roll it over your fillings. Tuck the top edge of the nori in and roll, using the parchment to press the roll tight. Repeat using the remaining nori sheets, sweet potatoes, and cucumber. Cut each roll into 8 equal pieces.

14. Sprinkle with the sesame seeds, and serve with garnishes of choice, such as soy sauce, wasabi, or pickled ginger.

PER SERVING (4 ROLLS): Calories: 838; Protein: 20g; Total fat: 26g; Carbohydrates: 138g; Fiber: 8g; Calcium: 160mg; Vitamin D: 0mg; Vitamin B_{12}: 0mg; Iron: 10mg; Zinc: 4mg

MACROS: Protein 7%; Carbs 66%; Fat 27%

TERIYAKI TOFU STIR-FRY

LOW-CARB

QUENCH THE HUNGER

RECOVERY BOOST

SERVES 3

PREP TIME: 20 minutes

COOK TIME: 15 minutes

FOR THE TERIYAKI SAUCE

¼ cup soy sauce, plus more
as needed

2 tablespoons chili-garlic
sauce or Sriracha sauce

2 tablespoons sesame oil

3 garlic cloves, minced

1 tablespoon coconut sugar
or sweetener of choice

1 tablespoon natural
peanut butter

1 tablespoon sesame seeds

FOR THE STIR-FRY

2 tablespoons olive
oil, divided

1 (16-ounce) block firm
tofu, drained, pressed,
and diced

1 medium red onion, cut
into thick slices

Stir-fry is a fantastic go-to on busy weekdays or when you need to quickly get something on the table. This dish is an excellent way to clear out any leftover vegetables in the crisper. The vegetables listed are just suggestions; feel free to use any that you like for this versatile recipe. Serve over a whole grain like brown rice or farro to balance the meal with all the nutrients you need.

TO MAKE THE TERIYAKI SAUCE

1. In a medium mixing bowl, whisk together the soy sauce, chili-garlic sauce, sesame oil, garlic, sugar, peanut butter, and sesame seeds. Adjust the seasoning with more soy sauce as needed.

TO MAKE THE STIR-FRY

2. In a large skillet, heat 1 tablespoon of olive oil over medium-high heat until it begins to shimmer.

3. Add the tofu and cook, tossing, for 5 to 6 minutes, until evenly golden brown on all sides. Transfer to the bowl with the teriyaki sauce.

4. In the same skillet, heat the remaining 1 tablespoon of olive oil over medium-high heat until it begins to shimmer.

5. Add the onion and sauté for 2 minutes or until it begins to soften.

6. Add the broccoli and carrots. Cook, tossing frequently, for 3 minutes.

1 small head broccoli, cut into florets

2 medium carrots, sliced on a bias

2 cups cremini (or any variety) mushrooms, quartered

1 small red bell pepper, cored and sliced

7. Add the mushrooms and bell pepper. Toss and cook for 2 to 3 minutes, until the vegetables are tender yet crisp.

8. Add the tofu and teriyaki sauce. Bring to a simmer, stirring until the sauce thickens slightly. Remove from the heat. Serve as is or over brown rice with a sprinkle of sesame seeds.

STORAGE: This is best eaten right away, but any leftovers can be refrigerated in a sealed container for up to 4 days.

SWAP IT: If you're pressed for time, use a store-bought teriyaki sauce; just be sure it contains whole-food ingredients.

PER SERVING: Calories: 432; Protein: 21g; Total fat: 32g; Carbohydrates: 21g; Fiber: 4g; Calcium: 313mg; Vitamin D: 2mg; Vitamin B$_{12}$: 0mg; Iron: 4mg; Zinc: 2mg

MACROS: Protein 17%; Carbs 19%; Fat 64%

BLACK BEAN AND QUINOA MEATBALLS WITH MARINARA SAUCE

SERVES 3

PREP TIME: 20 minutes, plus 15 minutes to chill

COOK TIME: 45 minutes

½ cup quinoa, rinsed

1 teaspoon sea salt, divided, plus more as needed

1 (15-ounce) can black beans, drained and rinsed

2 tablespoons olive oil or avocado oil, plus 1 teaspoon

1 small red onion, minced

3 garlic cloves, minced

1 teaspoon dried oregano

½ cup vegan Parmesan cheese

1 small bunch fresh basil leaves, coarsely chopped

2 tablespoons tomato paste

Freshly ground black pepper

2 cups store-bought marinara sauce

These simple, protein-packed vegan meatballs are sure to become a staple in your kitchen. The mixture can also be formed into patties for burgers or a loaf for a veggie "meat" loaf. Serve over high-protein pasta or on a sub roll for a heartier meal that will reload your glycogen stores.

1. Preheat the oven to 350°F. Line a baking sheet with parchment paper.

2. In a medium saucepan, combine 1½ cups water, the quinoa, and ½ teaspoon of salt. Bring to a boil over medium-high heat.

3. Reduce the heat to medium-low. Cover the saucepan and simmer for about 12 minutes, until the liquid has been absorbed. Remove from the heat. Let sit for 5 minutes, then uncover and fluff with a fork.

4. While the quinoa is cooking, spread the beans out in an even layer on the prepared baking sheet.

5. Transfer the baking sheet to the oven and cook for 10 to 12 minutes, until the beans have dried completely. Remove from the oven, leaving the oven on.

6. Increase the oven temperature to 375°F. Line another baking sheet with parchment paper.

7. In a large skillet, heat 2 tablespoons of oil over medium heat until it begins to shimmer. Add the onion, garlic, and remaining ½ teaspoon of salt. Sauté for 2 to 3 minutes, until slightly softened. Remove from the heat.

STORAGE: Refrigerate in an airtight container for up to 5 days, or freeze for up to 1 month.

SERVING TIP: These are great served over vegan pasta, rice, or vegetables, or on a toasted sandwich roll.

8. Put the beans, onion mixture, and oregano in a food processor. Pulse until just combined. Add the quinoa, cheese, basil, and tomato paste. Pulse until a firm dough forms. Adjust the seasoning with salt or pepper as needed.

9. Using a tablespoon, scoop out the mixture and roll it into balls with your hands. Place on the prepared baking sheet and refrigerate for 15 minutes.

10. In an oven-safe skillet, heat the remaining 1 teaspoon of oil over medium heat until it shimmers. Add the balls and cook, turning them to get a golden crust, for about 5 minutes. Remove from the heat.

11. Transfer the skillet to the oven and bake for about 20 minutes, until the balls are golden brown and firm to the touch. Remove from the oven.

12. Add the marinara sauce to the skillet and heat over medium heat for 5 minutes or until simmering and hot. Remove from the heat.

13. Serve the meatballs in warm bowls, with a sprinkle of additional cheese if desired.

PER SERVING: Calories: 443; Protein: 20g; Total fat: 17g; Carbohydrates: 55g; Fiber: 13g; Calcium: 223mg; Vitamin D: 4mg; Vitamin B_{12}: 0mg; Iron: 5mg; Zinc: 2mg

MACROS: Protein 16%; Carbs 48%; Fat 36%

GINGER AND GARLIC SEITAN

QUENCH THE HUNGER
RECOVERY BOOST

SERVES 4

PREP TIME: 10 minutes

COOK TIME: 20 minutes

2 tablespoons avocado
oil, divided

3 garlic cloves, minced

1 (1-inch) piece fresh
ginger, grated

½ teaspoon Chinese
five-spice powder

½ teaspoon red
pepper flakes

½ cup low-sodium
soy sauce

¼ cup coconut sugar or
sweetener of choice

3 teaspoons corn-
starch, divided

2 tablespoons cold water

1 pound Basic Seitan
(page 20) or
store-bought, cut into
1-inch dice

Toasted sesame seeds,
for serving

Sliced scallions, green and
white parts, for serving

This recipe is a great way to use Basic Seitan (page 20). The combination of crispy seitan and this sweet, salty, and slightly spicy sauce is positively addictive. Enjoy this dish with your favorite grain and a side of cooked vegetables. You can also add chopped vegetables to the pan with the seitan in step 9.

1. In a small skillet, heat 1 tablespoon of oil over medium heat until it begins to shimmer.

2. Add the garlic and ginger. Sauté for about 30 seconds.

3. Add the five-spice powder and red pepper flakes. Sauté for 30 seconds to release the aromas, being careful not to let the mixture burn.

4. Whisk in the soy sauce and sugar. Stir to combine.

5. Reduce the heat to low. Simmer for about 5 minutes, stirring occasionally, until the sugar has dissolved and the sauce has slightly reduced.

6. In a small bowl, whisk together 2 teaspoons of cornstarch and the cold water until completely combined. Stir into the skillet. Cook for about 2 minutes, until the sauce thickens slightly and appears glossy. Hold at a low simmer while cooking the seitan.

7. In a medium skillet, heat the remaining 1 tablespoon of oil over medium-high heat until it begins to shimmer.

8. While the oil is heating, in a bowl, toss the seitan lightly with the remaining 1 teaspoon of cornstarch.

9. Add the seitan to the skillet. Cook for about 5 minutes, tossing frequently, until golden brown and crispy.

10. Reduce the heat to low. Add the sauce to the skillet with the seitan. Toss to coat and cook for 1 to 2 minutes, until the sauce has caramelized. Remove from the heat.

11. Sprinkle with the sesame seeds and scallions. Enjoy the seitan on its own or with your favorite grain and vegetables.

STORAGE: Refrigerate in an airtight container for up to 4 days.

COOKING TIP: Seitan crisps nicely in an air fryer; just make the sauce in a large skillet and add the crisped seitan to the sauce to finish.

PER SERVING: Calories: 412; Protein: 46g; Total fat: 12g; Carbohydrates: 30g; Fiber: 2g; Calcium: 117mg; Vitamin D: 0mg; Vitamin B$_{12}$: 0mg; Iron: 5mg; Zinc: 1mg

MACROS: Protein 45%; Carbs 29%; Fat 26%

LEMON-ALMOND FETTUCCINE ALFREDO

HIGH-CARB

QUENCH THE HUNGER

SERVES 3

PREP TIME: 10 minutes

COOK TIME: 20 minutes

8 to 10 ounces fettuccine
or pasta of choice

3 tablespoons olive oil,
plus more for coating the
fettuccine

4 garlic cloves, minced

½ teaspoon sea salt, plus
more as needed

¼ cup all-purpose flour

2 cups unsweetened
almond milk

¼ cup Vegan Soft Cheese
(page 24) or vegan
Parmesan cheese, plus
more for serving

Grated zest and juice of
1 small lemon

1 teaspoon nutritional yeast

½ teaspoon garlic powder

Freshly ground
black pepper

1 cup fresh or frozen peas
(thawed if frozen)

Toasted sliced almonds, for
serving (optional)

This brightly flavored lemon alfredo comes together in just 30 minutes. It's a quick, creamy comfort dish that satisfies even the biggest appetites.

1. Bring a medium pot of water to a boil over high heat. Cook the fettuccine according to the package instructions. Drain, toss in a bit of oil to keep from sticking, and cover to keep warm.

2. Meanwhile, to make the sauce, in a large skillet, heat the oil over medium heat until it begins to shimmer.

3. Add the garlic and salt. Cook for about 30 seconds to release aromas.

4. Reduce the heat to medium-low. Add the flour and whisk to create a smooth roux. Cook, stirring, for about 1 minute.

5. While whisking quickly to prevent clumps, add the almond milk slowly in a thin stream. Cook, stirring occasionally, for 2 minutes. Remove from the heat. Transfer to a blender.

6. Add the cheese, lemon zest, lemon juice, nutritional yeast, and garlic powder. Blend on high speed, scraping down the sides as needed, until creamy and smooth. Adjust the seasoning with salt and pepper as needed.

7. Return the sauce to the skillet. Bring to a simmer over medium heat.

8. Reduce the heat to low. Cook for about 2 minutes, stirring frequently, until the sauce is thick and creamy. (You can add more milk as needed if the sauce is too thick.)

9. Add the fettuccine and peas. Toss to combine completely. Cook for 1 minute to warm through. Remove from the heat.

10. Serve the fettuccine in warm pasta bowls with a sprinkle of vegan cheese and toasted sliced almonds (if using).

STORAGE: Refrigerate in an airtight container for up to 4 days.

VARIATION: If you'd like to add extra protein to the pasta, toss in some diced tofu or seitan when you add the peas.

PER SERVING: Calories: 576; Protein: 21g; Total fat: 20g; Carbohydrates: 77g; Fiber: 6g; Calcium: 309mg; Vitamin D: 1mg; Vitamin B_{12}: 0mg; Iron: 2mg; Zinc: 2mg

MACROS: Protein 14%; Carbs 55%; Fat 31%

SPINACH AND TOFU ENCHILADAS WITH BLACK BEAN SAUCE

GLUTEN-FREE
NUT-FREE
QUENCH THE HUNGER
RECOVERY BOOST

Made with homemade sauce, tofu, and avocado oil, these enchiladas are just as gooey and cheesy as traditional versions, but with the health benefits of whole, protein-packed ingredients.

SERVES 4

PREP TIME: 20 minutes

COOK TIME: 40 to 45 minutes

FOR THE BLACK BEAN SAUCE

1 tablespoon whole black peppercorns

4 bay leaves

2 tablespoons avocado oil

½ onion, diced

1 teaspoon dried basil

1 teaspoon sea salt

1 cup canned black beans, drained and rinsed

FOR THE SAUTÉED SPINACH AND TOFU

1 tablespoon avocado oil

2 garlic cloves, minced

1 (16-ounce) block firm tofu, rinsed, drained, and cut into 1-inch cubes

1 (10-ounce) bag fresh baby spinach

TO MAKE THE BLACK BEAN SAUCE

1. Put the peppercorns and bay leaves in a large dry skillet over medium heat. Toast for about 30 seconds, until aromas are released. Remove the peppercorns and bay leaves from the skillet.

2. Pour the oil into the skillet and increase the heat to medium-high.

3. Add the onion, peppercorns, bay leaves, basil and salt. Sauté for about 3 minutes, until the onion is golden brown.

4. Add the beans and stir to combine. Remove from the heat. Let cool slightly. Working in batches, transfer the mixture to a blender, and blend with a little water as needed to achieve a sauce consistency. It should be smooth and velvety.

5. Pour the sauce into a pot. Cover and place on a burner over the lowest heat to keep warm.

TO MAKE THE SAUTÉED SPINACH AND TOFU

6. In a medium skillet, heat the oil over medium heat until it shimmers.

7. Add the garlic and sauté for 1 minute or until translucent.

FOR THE ENCHILADAS

12 (6-inch) blue or white corn tortillas

2 ripe avocados, pitted, peeled, and sliced

1 cup shredded vegan cheese of choice

STORAGE: Refrigerate the sauce in an airtight container for up to 1 week, or freeze for up to 6 months.

SWAP IT: Use any kind of vegetables you like in these enchiladas; they're a great way to use up trimmings or leftovers.

8. Add the tofu and sauté for about 5 minutes, until golden.

9. Add the spinach and sauté for about 1 minute, until wilted. Remove from the heat.

TO MAKE THE ENCHILADAS

10. Preheat the oven to 375°F.

11. Warm the tortillas in the microwave for about 30 seconds, until soft.

12. Pour the sauce into a large baking or casserole dish. Dip 1 tortilla in the sauce, then add a spoonful of the spinach-tofu mixture to the tortilla and spread it out evenly.

13. Add a few slices of avocado.

14. Cover the filling with another tortilla dipped in black bean sauce. Repeat with the remaining sauce, tortillas, spinach-tofu mixture, and avocados.

15. Cover the enchiladas with the cheese.

16. Transfer the baking dish to the oven and bake for 30 minutes or until the cheese is bubbly and brown. Remove from the oven and serve.

PER SERVING: Calories: 669; Protein: 28g; Total fat: 38g; Carbohydrates: 72g; Fiber: 18g; Calcium: 514mg; Vitamin D: 0mg; Vitamin B$_{12}$: 0mg; Iron: 7mg; Zinc: 4mg

MACROS: Protein 15%; Carbs 39%; Fat 46%

GNOCCHI WITH CHICKPEAS AND BASIL-WALNUT PESTO

HIGH-CARB

QUENCH THE HUNGER

SERVES 3

PREP TIME: 10 minutes

COOK TIME: 10 minutes

4 ounces fresh basil (about
   2 cups packed leaves)

¼ cup coarsely
   chopped walnuts

½ cup olive oil, divided

1 garlic clove, peeled
   and smashed

1 teaspoon freshly
   squeezed lemon juice

Sea salt

Freshly ground
   black pepper

1 cup raw cashews

1 cup water, plus more
   as needed

1 (15-ounce) can chickpeas,
   drained and rinsed

1 pound gnocchi

> **VARIATION:** For a more vegetable-forward gnocchi, swap the chickpeas for peas and asparagus.

Gnocchi gets a vegan makeover here—and is ideal after a hard day of training. The chickpeas and walnuts provide protein, and the pesto brings healthy fats along with the flavor.

1. To make the pesto, put the basil, walnuts, ¼ cup of oil, the garlic, and lemon juice in a food processor. Pulse just until everything is combined and the pesto retains some of its texture.

2. While continuing to pulse, add the remaining ¼ cup of oil through the chute in the processor lid. Adjust the seasoning with salt and pepper as needed.

3. To make the cashew cream, put the cashews and water in a high-speed blender. Blend until very smooth, adding a little more water for texture and scraping down the sides as needed.

4. Pour the cashew cream into a large skillet over medium-low heat. Whisk in the pesto, and add the chickpeas and gnocchi. Cook for 2 to 3 minutes, stirring occasionally, until heated through. Remove from the heat. Serve immediately.

STORAGE: Refrigerate in an airtight container for up to 3 days, or freeze for up to 2 months.

PER SERVING: Calories: 986; Protein: 23g; Total fat: 75g; Carbohydrates: 65g; Fiber: 11g; Calcium: 168mg; Vitamin D: 15mg; Vitamin B$_{12}$: 0mg; Iron: 8mg; Zinc: 5mg

MACROS: Protein 9%; Carbs 26%; Fat 65%

SMOKY LENTIL CHORIZO TACOS

GLUTEN-FREE
HIGH-CARB
QUENCH THE HUNGER
RECOVERY BOOST

This walnut-lentil chorizo is super flavorful and packed with protein, omegas, and fiber. In addition to tacos, it makes an excellent filling for burritos or a great topping for a grain bowl.

SERVES 4

PREP TIME: 10 minutes
COOK TIME: 25 minutes

1 cup dried green lentils
3 cups water
Pinch sea salt, plus
 1 teaspoon
1¼ cups walnut pieces,
 coarsely chopped
½ cup sun-dried tomatoes,
 coarsely chopped
1 tablespoon
 smoked paprika
2 teaspoons garlic powder
1 teaspoon chili powder
1 teaspoon dried oregano
½ teaspoon ground cumin
½ teaspoon dried thyme
¼ teaspoon ground
 cinnamon
¼ teaspoon red pepper
 flakes (optional)
12 (4-inch) corn torti-
 llas, warmed

1. In a medium saucepan, combine the lentils, water, and pinch of salt. Bring to a boil over medium-high heat.

2. Reduce the heat to low. Simmer for 15 to 20 minutes, until the lentils are just tender. Remove from the heat.

3. Meanwhile, put the walnuts, sun-dried tomatoes, paprika, garlic powder, chili powder, remaining 1 teaspoon of salt, oregano, cumin, thyme, cinnamon, and red pepper flakes (if using) in a food processor.

4. When the lentils are cooked, drain them in a fine-mesh strainer, then add them to the food processor. Pulse until the mixture resembles a moist crumble.

5. Spoon the mixture into the tortillas, and serve immediately.

STORAGE: Store in an airtight container in the refrigerator for up to 5 days, or freeze for up to 2 months.

PER SERVING (3 TACOS): Calories: 566; Protein: 22g; Total fat: 27g; Carbohydrates: 65g; Fiber: 13g; Calcium: 166mg; Vitamin D: 0mg; Vitamin B_{12}: 0mg; Iron: 7mg; Zinc: 4mg

MACROS: Protein 15%; Carbs 44%; Fat 41%

VEGAN POWER PIZZA

HIGH-CARB

QUENCH THE HUNGER

RECOVERY BOOST

MAKES 1 LARGE PIZZA

PREP TIME: 10 minutes, plus 30 minutes to rest

COOK TIME: 15 minutes

1 cup warm water

1 packet fast-acting yeast

2 tablespoons sugar, divided

1 cup all-purpose flour, plus more for dusting

¼ cup chickpea flour

¼ cup Pea Protein Powder (page 18) or store-bought protein powder

1 teaspoon sea salt, plus more as needed

½ teaspoon garlic powder

2 tablespoons olive oil, plus more for brushing

½ cup store-bought marinara sauce

½ cup Vegan Soft Cheese (page 24)

¼ cup cooked seitan bacon, crumbled

½ cup fresh basil leaves, chopped

This easy-to-make vegan pie has a delicious, pillowy crust that tops delivery pizza any day, and it's one of my favorite ways to use up leftover vegetables. Play around with your favorite toppings, or use the ones I suggest here. If you don't have chickpea flour, use ½ cup all-purpose flour instead.

1. In a small bowl, stir together the warm water, yeast, and ½ tablespoon of sugar until dissolved. Let sit for about 10 minutes to activate the yeast; it should begin to foam.

2. In a large bowl, whisk together the all-purpose flour, chickpea flour, protein powder, salt, garlic powder, and remaining 1½ tablespoons of sugar.

3. Whisk in the yeast mixture and oil. Mix until all the ingredients are well combined and form a dough.

4. Using your hands, roll the dough into a ball, then place it back in the bowl. Cover the bowl with a clean, damp towel; set aside in a warm spot for 30 minutes or until the dough doubles in size.

5. Preheat the oven to 500°F. Line a baking sheet with a piece of parchment paper.

6. Dust the parchment with a bit of flour, and, using your hands, press out the dough across the parchment into your favorite pizza shape and desired thickness. Pinch the edges up slightly, or leave the crust flat if you prefer. Brush the dough lightly with a little oil, and sprinkle with salt.

7. Using a large spoon, spread the sauce evenly over the pizza.

8. Top with the cheese, and sprinkle with the bacon.

9. Place the pizza on the middle oven rack, and bake for 10 to 15 minutes, until the crust is golden brown. Remove from the oven.

10. Sprinkle with the basil, slice, and serve hot.

STORAGE: Refrigerate in an airtight container for up to 5 days, or freeze for up to 1 month.

MAKE AHEAD: I like to double the recipe, bake an extra crust, and keep it in the freezer for a super-quick pizza night.

PER SERVING (¼ PIZZA): Calories: 385; Protein: 21g; Total fat: 13g; Carbohydrates: 47g; Fiber: 4g; Calcium: 147mg; Vitamin D: 0mg; Vitamin B$_{12}$: 0mg; Iron: 5mg; Zinc: 2mg

MACROS: Protein 21%; Carbs 49%; Fat 30%

CHICKPEA "CRAB" CAKES

HIGH-CARB

NUT-FREE

QUENCH THE HUNGER

RECOVERY BOOST

MAKES 8 CRAB CAKES

PREP TIME: 15 minutes

COOK TIME: 10 minutes

1 (15-ounce) can chickpeas, drained, rinsed, and dried

1 (14-ounce) can quartered artichoke hearts, rinsed and dried

1 large red bell pepper, cored and coarsely chopped

1 scallion, green and white parts, coarsely chopped

1 celery stalk, coarsely chopped

½ small bunch fresh parsley, coarsely chopped, or 1 tablespoon dried parsley

1½ cups panko bread crumbs, divided

3 tablespoons Vegan Mayonnaise (page 25)

3 tablespoons chickpea flour or ¼ cup all-purpose flour

2 tablespoons whole-grain mustard

These chickpea cakes are so simple to make. Just throw everything in a food processor, shape it into cakes, and pan-fry. They are a guaranteed crowd-pleaser and make-ahead friendly.

1. Put the chickpeas and artichoke hearts in a food processor. Pulse 3 or 4 times to just combine, but don't overprocess. The mixture should be chunky. Transfer to a large mixing bowl.

2. Put the bell pepper, scallion, celery, and parsley in the food processor. Process until minced, scraping down the sides of the food processor bowl as needed, and then add this mixture to the chickpea mixture.

3. Fold in 1 cup of bread crumbs, the mayonnaise, chickpea flour, mustard, Old Bay seasoning, salt, cayenne, and lemon juice. Mix thoroughly until well combined. The mixture should hold together when pressed.

4. Line a baking sheet with parchment paper. Pack some of the "crab" cake mixture into a ¼-cup measure, then tap the cup gently to release the cake onto the baking sheet. Repeat to make 8 cakes total.

5. Put the remaining ½ cup of bread crumbs on a plate, dredge the cakes in them, and return the cakes to the baking sheet.

6. In a heavy or cast-iron skillet, heat ¼ inch of oil over medium heat until it shimmers.

2 teaspoons Old Bay
seasoning

1 teaspoon sea salt, plus
more as needed

¼ teaspoon cay-
enne pepper

Juice of 1 lemon

Avocado oil, for frying

Vegan tartar sauce, for
serving (optional)

Lemon wedges, for serving

7. Using a spatula, gently place the "crab" cakes in the skillet. Cook for 3 to 4 minutes per side, until golden and crispy. Remove from the heat. Transfer to warm plates. Sprinkle with a bit of salt.

8. Serve the cakes with tartar sauce (if using) and lemon wedges.

STORAGE: Refrigerate in an airtight container for up to 5 days, or freeze for up to 2 months. The cakes can also be frozen before cooking for up to 3 months, or you can prep them 1 day in advance, store the uncooked cakes in an airtight container in the refrigerator, and cook them the next day.

SERVING TIP: Mini "crab" cakes make for great party hors d'oeuvres; they are also fantastic on toasted English muffins as the classic East Coast sandwiches.

PER SERVING (2 CAKES): Calories: 608; Protein: 27g; Total fat: 18g; Carbohydrates: 85g; Fiber: 21g; Calcium: 141mg; Vitamin D: 0mg; Vitamin B_{12}: 0mg; Iron: 7mg; Zinc: 4mg

MACROS: Protein 18%; Carbs 56%; Fat 26%

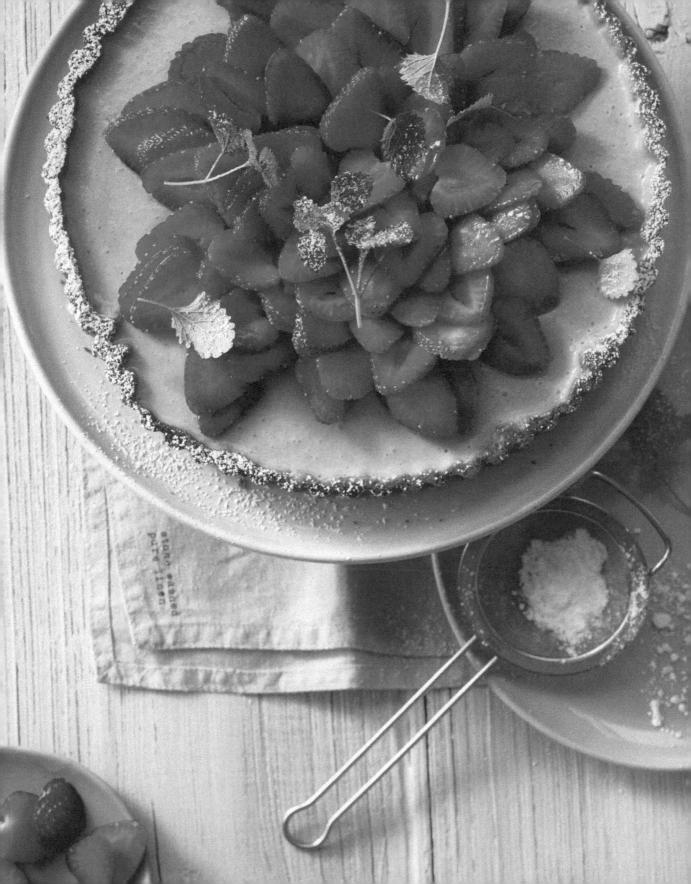

7

DESSERTS

Dessert matters to me. I have a sweet tooth and couldn't imagine life without a little dessert goodness. In a vegan lifestyle, it can be challenging to find dessert recipes that are easy to make at home, deliver on delicious, and provide good nutrition to support your lifestyle. In this chapter, you'll find recipe solutions that make dessert accessible for you. Not all the recipes are high in protein, but they all contain a source of plant-based protein to help top off your needs for the day. They are also so tasty that you'll want to share them with everyone.

Strawberry Cheesecake
page 122

VANILLA COCONUT YOGURT PANNA COTTA

GLUTEN-FREE

HIGH-CARB

NUT-FREE

RECOVERY BOOST

SERVES 6

PREP TIME: 20 minutes, plus 2 hours to set

3 tablespoons plant-based gelatin, such as agar powder

6 tablespoons cold water

3 cups unsweetened vanilla coconut milk yogurt

2 tablespoons monk fruit sweetener or sweetener of choice, plus more as needed

1 vanilla bean, split and scraped, or 2 teaspoons vanilla extract

2 cups diced fruit or berries of choice

½ cup toasted unsweet-ened shredded coconut

VARIATION: This panna cotta is equally good with a mixture of tropical fruits or berries; for extra protein and crunch, add some toasted walnuts.

This coconut panna cotta is perfect when you want a fuss-free dessert. I like monk fruit sweet-ener here but any kind of sugar will work.

1. In a small mixing bowl, whisk together the gelatin and cold water until well combined. Set aside for about 10 minutes, until set.

2. Meanwhile, in a large mixing bowl, whisk together the coconut yogurt, monk fruit sweetener, and vanilla.

3. Melt the set gelatin mixture in a microwave on high power for about 10 seconds or in a hot water bath.

4. Add the melted gelatin mixture to the coconut yogurt mixture, and whisk together for 30 seconds. Adjust the flavor with a little more sweetener as needed.

5. Divide the mixture among 6 (4-ounce) glass ramekins or small glasses. Place the ramekins on a small baking sheet, and cover with plastic wrap. Refrigerate for at least 2 hours to set completely. The panna cotta should be firm but will still jiggle a little when tapped.

6. Top with the fruit and coconut flakes.

STORAGE: Refrigerate in an airtight container for up to 10 days.

PER SERVING: Calories: 170; Protein: 5g; Total fat: 5g; Carbohydrates: 27g; Fiber: 2g; Calcium: 165mg; Vitamin D: 0mg; Vitamin B$_{12}$: 0mg; Iron: 2mg; Zinc: 1mg

MACROS: Protein 13%; Carbs 63%; Fat 24%

BANANA, ALMOND BUTTER, AND CHIA PUDDING

SERVES 2

PREP TIME: 5 minutes, plus
2 hours to set

2 cups unsweetened
   almond milk

6 tablespoons
   almond butter

2 bananas, cut into
   large chunks

2 teaspoons pure
   maple syrup

1 teaspoon ground
   cinnamon

½ teaspoon sea salt

6 tablespoons chia seeds

This is another quick and easy dessert that you can feel good about eating any time of day, even for breakfast! It's a powerhouse pudding packed with protein and fiber, and it's just sweet enough to be a treat. If possible, use Ceylon cinnamon here. It is a powerful antioxidant and immune system booster, along with being a blood sugar stabilizer.

1. Put the almond milk, almond butter, bananas, maple syrup, cinnamon, and salt in a high-speed blender or food processor. Process for about 30 seconds, until the ingredients are completely combined. Pour into a medium glass bowl or jar.

2. Stir in the chia seeds and refrigerate for at least 2 hours or overnight.

3. Serve as is, or top with toasted almonds, sliced fruit, berries, or additional almond butter.

STORAGE: Refrigerate in an airtight container for up to 2 days.

VARIATION: This dessert is equally delicious made with any nut butter; I really love it with walnut butter.

PER SERVING: Calories: 723; Protein: 26g; Total fat: 44g; Carbohydrates: 67g; Fiber: 25g; Calcium: 761mg; Vitamin D: 0mg; Vitamin B$_{12}$: 3mg; Iron: 7mg; Zinc: 4mg

MACROS: Protein 13%; Carbs 35%; Fat 52%

DARK CHERRY AND CHOCOLATE ICE CREAM

GLUTEN-FREE

LOW-CARB

NUT-FREE

RECOVERY BOOST

SERVES 4

PREP TIME: 20 minutes, plus at least 6 hours to freeze

¾ cup water or cherry juice

1¼ cups coconut milk

¾ cup cocoa powder

½ cup coconut sugar or sweetener of choice

⅛ teaspoon sea salt

1½ cups dark cherries, pitted and diced

4 ounces dark chocolate, chopped

VARIATION: For a little extra decadence, I like to add 1 teaspoon cherry brandy to this in step 2; it also helps prevent ice crystals from forming, especially if you are not using an ice cream maker.

Dark chocolate–covered cherries are a match made in dessert heaven—and my biggest weakness when it comes to sweets. I adore them so much that my mother sends me a box for my birthday every year. I came up with this ice cream to satisfy my craving. This version is lightly sweetened and enhanced with the antioxidant power of dark cherries and chocolate, great for recovery. If you don't have an ice cream maker, freeze the mixture in the baking dish.

1. In a small saucepan, bring the water and coconut milk to a boil.

2. Whisk in the cocoa powder, sugar, and salt. Stir until dissolved. Remove from the heat.

3. Pour the mixture into a 3-quart glass baking dish, and refrigerate until very cold.

4. Pour the mixture into an ice cream maker, and process according to the manufacturer's instructions. Pour the ice cream into a medium bowl.

5. Fold in the cherries and dark chocolate. Serve immediately, or cover and freeze until ready to serve.

STORAGE: Store in an airtight container in the freezer for up to 2 months.

PER SERVING: Calories: 474; Protein: 7g; Total fat: 29g; Carbohydrates: 57g; Fiber: 9g; Calcium: 64mg; Vitamin D: 0mg; Vitamin B$_{12}$: 0mg; Iron: 8mg; Zinc: 2mg

MACROS: Protein 4%; Carbs 42%; Fat 54%

RASPBERRY–BLACK BEAN CHOCOLATE MOUSSE

GLUTEN-FREE

QUENCH THE HUNGER

SERVES 4

PREP TIME: 5 minutes, plus 2 hours to chill

1 (15-ounce) can black beans, drained and rinsed

½ cup unsweetened almond milk

¼ cup cocoa powder

¼ cup pure maple syrup

3 tablespoons raw cashews

2 tablespoons coconut butter or any nut butter

⅛ teaspoon sea salt

⅛ teaspoon ground cinnamon

6 ounces fresh or frozen raspberries (thawed if frozen)

Mousse made with black beans? You read that right! The black beans give this mousse a creamy texture and pack some protein into this rich dessert. But don't worry, you won't taste them. This mousse is deeply chocolatey with a touch of naturally sweet maple syrup.

1. Put the beans, almond milk, cocoa powder, maple syrup, cashews, coconut butter, salt, and cinnamon in a high-speed blender or food processor. Blend until very smooth. Spoon into 4 (4-ounce) glass ramekins or glasses.

2. Arrange the raspberries on top. Refrigerate for at least 2 hours.

STORAGE: Refrigerate in an airtight container for up to 1 week.

SWAP IT: Any kind of fruit works well here. Or try peanut butter for a chocolate–peanut butter mousse.

PER SERVING: Calories: 271; Protein: 11g; Total fat: 10g; Carbohydrates: 41g; Fiber: 11g; Calcium: 123mg; Vitamin D: 0mg; Vitamin B$_{12}$: 0mg; Iron: 3mg; Zinc: 2mg

MACROS: Protein 14%; Carbs 56%; Fat 30%

STRAWBERRY CHEESECAKE

MAKES 1 (6-INCH) ROUND CAKE

PREP TIME: 30 minutes, plus 1 hour to soak and 4 hours to freeze

2 cups raw cashews

¼ cup coconut oil, melted and cooled, plus 2 teaspoons for greasing

1 cup shredded coconut

½ cup pecan pieces

6 pitted dates

¼ teaspoon sea salt

½ cup canned coconut milk, shaken, plus more as needed

⅓ cup pure maple syrup

2 tablespoons freshly squeezed lemon juice

1 teaspoon vanilla extract

1 pint fresh or frozen strawberries (thawed if frozen), halved, divided

2 teaspoons coconut sugar or sweetener of choice

If you think cheesecake can't be vegan, think again. This rich and creamy version is the perfect dessert to serve at a dinner party, and it delivers on all things cheesecake. As a bonus, two types of nuts are used to provide a small dose of plant-based protein, too.

1. Put the cashews in a mixing bowl with enough boiling water to cover them by 1 inch. Let soak for 1 hour.

2. Meanwhile, grease a 6-inch springform pan with 2 teaspoons of coconut oil.

3. Put the shredded coconut, pecans, dates, and salt in a food processor. Process until a dough forms. Press the dough evenly onto the bottom of the prepared springform pan.

4. Put the coconut milk, maple syrup, remaining ¼ cup of coconut oil, the lemon juice, vanilla, and ¼ cup of strawberries in a blender. Blend for about 2 minutes, until the mixture is very smooth, adding a bit more coconut milk as needed.

5. Pour the coconut milk mixture over the dough in the pan. Freeze for at least 4 hours, until completely set.

6. While the cheesecake is freezing, make the compote: In a small saucepan, combine the remaining strawberries and the sugar. Bring to a boil over medium heat.

7. Reduce the heat to low. Cook until the strawberries release their liquid to create a syrup. Remove from the heat. Let cool completely until ready to serve.

8. Let the cheesecake thaw for about 15 minutes at room temperature, then slice and serve it with the compote on top.

STORAGE: Refrigerate in an airtight container for up to 5 days, or freeze for up to 2 months.

SWAP IT: Cheesecake works with all fruits as a topping; try eating this with blueberries or cherries. If compote's not your jam, you can also top this with fresh strawberries, a little powdered sugar, and a sprig of mint.

PER SERVING (⅛ CAKE): Calories: 446; Protein: 9g; Total fat: 35g; Carbohydrates: 32g; Fiber: 4g; Calcium: 46mg; Vitamin D: 0mg; Vitamin B$_{12}$: 0mg; Iron: 4mg; Zinc: 3mg

MACROS: Protein 7%; Carbs 27%; Fat 66%

VEGAN DARK CHOCOLATE PROTEIN PUDDING

SERVES 2

PREP TIME: 5 minutes, plus
1 hour to chill

1 cup unsweetened
    almond milk
3 tablespoons chia seeds
1 scoop (2 tablespoons)
    Pea Protein Powder
    (page 18) or store-bought
    chocolate protein powder
2 tablespoons pure
    maple syrup
1 tablespoon cocoa powder
¼ teaspoon sea salt

*This vegan version of a classic comfort dessert
pudding is just as rich, silky, and creamy as the
original. It's a real treat for breakfast, a snack, or a
healthy dessert.*

Put the almond milk, chia seeds, protein powder, maple
syrup, cocoa powder, and salt in a high-speed blender.
Blend on high speed for about 1 minute, until completely smooth. Pour into 2 (6-ounce) glasses or jars,
and refrigerate for at least 1 hour or overnight before
serving.

STORAGE: Refrigerate in an airtight container for up
to 3 days.

SERVING TIP: Top with tropical fruits, berries, cacao nibs,
coconut, chopped nuts, coconut whipped cream, or chocolate chips.

PER SERVING: Calories: 289; Protein: 20g; Total fat: 10g;
Carbohydrates: 32g; Fiber: 10g; Calcium: 347mg; Vitamin D: 0mg;
Vitamin B$_{12}$: 1mg; Iron: 5mg; Zinc: 3mg

MACROS: Protein 27%; Carbs 43%; Fat 30%

MEASUREMENT CONVERSIONS

VOLUME EQUIVALENTS	U.S. STANDARD	U.S. STANDARD (OUNCES)	METRIC (APPROXIMATE)
LIQUID	2 tablespoons	1 fl. oz.	30 mL
	¼ cup	2 fl. oz.	60 mL
	½ cup	4 fl. oz.	120 mL
	1 cup	8 fl. oz.	240 mL
	1½ cups	12 fl. oz.	355 mL
	2 cups or 1 pint	16 fl. oz.	475 mL
	4 cups or 1 quart	32 fl. oz.	1 L
	1 gallon	128 fl. oz.	4 L
DRY	⅛ teaspoon		0.5 mL
	¼ teaspoon		1 mL
	½ teaspoon		2 mL
	¾ teaspoon		4 mL
	1 teaspoon		5 mL
	1 tablespoon		15 mL
	¼ cup		59 mL
	⅓ cup		79 mL
	½ cup		118 mL
	⅔ cup		156 mL
	¾ cup		177 mL
	1 cup		235 mL
	2 cups or 1 pint		475 mL
	3 cups		700 mL
	4 cups or 1 quart		1 L
	½ gallon		2 L
	1 gallon		4 L

OVEN TEMPERATURES

FAHRENHEIT	CELSIUS (APPROXIMATE)
250°F	120°C
300°F	150°C
325°F	165°C
350°F	180°C
375°F	190°C
400°F	200°C
425°F	220°C
450°F	230°C

WEIGHT EQUIVALENTS

U.S. STANDARD	METRIC (APPROXIMATE)
½ ounce	15 g
1 ounce	30 g
2 ounces	60 g
4 ounces	115 g
8 ounces	225 g
12 ounces	340 g
16 ounces or 1 pound	455 g

RESOURCES

- Academy of Nutrition and Dietetics's Find a Nutrition Expert: EatRight.org /find-a-nutrition-expert

- Sports nutrition for teen athletes: OffSeasonAthlete.com

- Sprouted Flour Company (sprouted grains, flours, and beans): HealthyFlour.com

- Healthy, organic foods and vegan specialties: ThriveMarket.com

- Asian ingredients: HMart.com

- Latin American ingredients: MexGrocer.com

- Mediterranean, Middle Eastern, and Indian spices: Kalustyans.com

- Sustainable produce and more: ImperfectFoods.com

REFERENCES

Babault, Nicolas, Christos Païzis, Gaëlle Deley, Laetitia Guérin-Deremaux, Marie-Hélène Saniez, Catherine Lefranc-Millot, and François A. Allaert. "Pea Proteins Oral Supplementation Promotes Muscle Thickness Gains during Resistance Training: A Double-Blind, Randomized, Placebo-Controlled Clinical Trial versus Whey Protein." *Journal of the International Society of Sports Nutrition* 12 (2015): 3. doi.org/10.1186/s12970-014-0064-5.

Berrazaga, Insaf, Valérie Micard, Marine Gueugneau, and Stéphane Walrand. "The Role of the Anabolic Properties of Plant- versus Animal-Based Protein Sources in Supporting Muscle Mass Maintenance: A Critical Review." *Nutrients* 11, no. 8 (August 2019): 1825. doi.org/10.3390/nu11081825.

Bosland, Maarten C., Jonathan Huang, Michael J. Schlicht, Erika Enk, Hui Xie, and Ikuko Kato. "Impact of 18-Month Soy Protein Supplementation on Steroid Hormones and Serum Biomarkers of Angiogenesis, Apoptosis, and the Growth Hormone/IGF-1 Axis: Results of a Randomized, Placebo-Controlled Trial in Males Following Prostatectomy." *Nutrition and Cancer* (2021). tandfonline.com/doi/abs/10.1080/01635581.2020.1870706.

Duitama, Sandra M., Javier Zurita, Diana Cordoba, Paola Duran, Leopold Ilag, and Wilson Mejia. "Soy Protein Supplement Intake for 12 Months Has No Effect on Sexual Maturation and May Improve Nutritional Status in Pre-Pubertal Children." *Journal of Paediatrics and Child Health* 54, no. 9 (September 2018): 997–1004. doi.org/10.1111/jpc.13934.

Fuhrman, Joel, and Deana M. Ferreri. "Fueling the Vegetarian (Vegan) Athlete." *Current Sports Medicine Reports* 9, no. 4 (July/August 2010): 233–41. doi.org/10.1249/JSR.0b013e3181e93a6f.

Hector, Amy J., and Stuart M. Phillips. "Protein Recommendations for Weight Loss in Elite Athletes: A Focus on Body Composition and Performance." *International Journal of Sport Nutrition and Exercise Metabolism* 28, no. 2 (2018): 170–77. doi.org/10.1123/ijsnem.2017-0273.

Iraki, Juma, Peter Fitschen, Sergio Espinar, and Eric Helms. "Nutrition Recommendations for Bodybuilders in the Off-Season: A Narrative Review." *Sports* 7, no. 7 (2019): 154. doi.org/10.3390/sports7070154.

Ji, Xiao-Jun, Lu-Jing Ren, and He Huang. "Omega-3 Biotechnology: A Green and Sustainable Process for Omega-3 Fatty Acids Production." *Frontiers in Bioengineering and Biotechnology* 3 (2015): 158. doi.org/10.3389/fbioe.2015.00158.

Karpinski, Christine, and Christine A. Rosenbloom. *Sports Nutrition: A Handbook for Professionals*. 6th ed. Chicago: Academy of Nutrition and Dietetics, 2017.

Loenneke, Jeremy P., Paul D. Loprinzi, Caoileann H. Murphy, and Stuart M. Phillips. "Per Meal Dose and Frequency of Protein Consumption Is Associated with Lean Mass and Muscle Performance." *Clinical Nutrition* 35, no. 6 (2016): 1506–11. doi.org/10.1016/j.clnu.2016.04.002.

Lynch, Heidi, Carol Johnston, and Christopher Wharton. "Plant-Based Diets: Considerations for Environmental Impact, Protein Quality, and Exercise Performance." *Nutrients* 10, no. 12 (December 2018): 1841. doi.org/10.3390/nu10121841.

Messina, Mark, Heidi Lynch, Jared M. Dickinson, and Katharine E. Reed. "No Difference between the Effects of Supplementing with Soy Protein versus Animal Protein on Gains in Muscle Mass and Strength in Response to Resistance Exercise." *International Journal of Sport Nutrition and Exercise Metabolism* 28, no. 6 (2018): 674–85. doi.org/10.1123/ijsnem.2018-0071.

Mobley, C. Brooks, Cody T. Haun, Paul A. Roberson, Petey W. Mumford, Matthew A. Romero, Wesley C. Kephart, Richard G. Anderson, et al. "Effects of Whey, Soy or Leucine Supplementation with 12 Weeks of Resistance Training on Strength, Body Composition, and Skeletal Muscle and Adipose Tissue Histological Attributes in College-Aged Males." *Nutrients* 9, no. 9 (2017): 972. doi.org/10.3390/nu9090972.

Moore, Daniel R., Donny M. Camera, Jose L. Areta, and John A. Hawley. "Beyond Muscle Hypertrophy: Why Dietary Protein Is Important for Endurance Athletes." *Applied Physiology, Nutrition, and Metabolism* 39, no. 9 (2014): 987–97. doi.org/10.1139/apnm-2013-0591.

Morrell, P, and S. Fiszman. "Revisiting the Role of Protein-Induced Satiation and Satiety." *Food Hydrocolloids* 68 (July 2017): 199–210. doi.org/10.1016/j.foodhyd.2016.08.003.

Nagao, Takayo, and Makato Hirokawa. "Diagnosis and Treatment of Macrocytic Anemias in Adults." *Journal of General and Family Medicine* 18, no. 5 (2017): 200–204. doi.org/10.1002/jgf2.31.

National Center for Biotechnology Information. "PubChem Compound Summary: Histidine, CID 6274." Accessed Feb. 20, 2021. pubchem.ncbi.nlm.nih.gov/compound/Histidine.

National Center for Biotechnology Information. "PubChem Compound Summary: I-Isoleucine, CID 6306." Accessed Feb. 20, 2021. pubchem.ncbi.nlm.nih.gov/compound/isoleucine.

National Center for Biotechnology Information. "PubChem Compound Summary: L-Threonine, CID 6288." Accessed Feb. 20, 2021. pubchem.ncbi.nlm.nih.gov/compound/L-Threonine.

National Center for Biotechnology Information. "PubChem Compound Summary: Leucine, CID 6106." Accessed Feb. 20, 2021. pubchem.ncbi.nlm.nih.gov/compound/Leucine.

National Center for Biotechnology Information. "PubChem Compound Summary: Lysine, CID 5962." Accessed Feb. 20, 2021. pubchem.ncbi.nlm.nih.gov/compound/Lysine.

National Center for Biotechnology Information. "PubChem Compound Summary: Methionine, CID 6137." Accessed Feb. 20, 2021. pubchem.ncbi.nlm.nih.gov/compound/Methionine.

National Center for Biotechnology Information. "PubChem Compound Summary: Phenylalanine, CID 6140." Accessed Feb. 20, 2021. pubchem.ncbi.nlm.nih.gov/compound/Phenylalanine.

National Center for Biotechnology Information. "PubChem Compound Summary: Tryptophan, CID 6305."
Accessed Feb. 20, 2021. pubchem.ncbi.nlm.nih.gov/compound/Tryptophan.

National Center for Biotechnology Information. "PubChem Compound Summary: Valine, CID 6287."
Accessed Feb. 20, 2021. pubchem.ncbi.nlm.nih.gov/compound/Valine.

Segovia-Siapco, Gina, Peter Pribis, Keiji Oda, and Joan Sabaté. "Soy Isoflavone Consumption and Age at
Pubarche in Adolescent Males." *European Journal of Nutrition* 57 (2018): 2287–94. doi.org/10.1007
/s00394-017-1504-1.

Shenoy, Shweta, Mrinal Dhawan, and Jaspal Singh Sandhu. "Four Weeks of Supplementation with Isolated
Soy Protein Attenuates Exercise-Induced Muscle Damage and Enhances Muscle Recovery in Well
Trained Athletes: A Randomized Trial." *Asian Journal of Sports Medicine* 7, no. 3 (2016): e33528.
doi.org/10.5812/asjsm.33528.

Thomas, D. Travis, Kelly Anne Erdman, and Louise M. Burke. "Position of the Academy of Nutrition and
Dietetics, Dietitians of Canada, and the American College of Sports Medicine: Nutrition and Athletic
Performance." *Journal of the Academy of Nutrition and Dietetics* 116, no. 3 (2016): 501–28. doi.org
/10.1016/j.jand.2015.12.006.

Zhang, Shihai, Xiangfang Zeng, Man Ren, Xiangbing Mao, and Shiyan Qiao. "Novel Metabolic and
Physiological Functions of Branched Chain Amino Acids: A Review." *Journal of Animal Science and
Biotechnology* 8 (2017): 10. doi.org/10.1186/s40104-016-0139-z.

INDEX

H

Acknowledgments

JENNA: From the day I became a dietitian in 2005, I knew I wanted to work with athletes. Although I don't consider myself a gifted athlete, it is my greatest joy to see someone perform at their best due to a strong nutrition plan. I've been blessed to work with a plethora of tremendous athletes, from very young gymnasts to master rowers. Thank you to all these athletes (and parents) who trusted me to walk alongside them as they pursued their goals. I've learned from each of these relationships, and that has helped shape me into the sports dietitian I am today.

To the many mentors I've had in my career, thank you for investing in me. Sports nutrition is a discipline that requires you to learn from others, and I'm so grateful for the many people who have been willing to teach me.

Thank you, Ivy, for being such a wonderful partner on this project. I am in awe of your expertise and talent, and I'm so glad this book brought us together.

To my family, Brian, Jackson, and Benjamin: I love you deeply and am so thankful for you. I look forward to watching my favorite coach and two favorite athletes grow and achieve in the years to come.

May God be glorified through the work He has given me to do. "For from him and through him and for him are all things. To him be the glory forever! Amen" (Romans 11:36).

IVY: I would like to thank the team of collaborators on this book, first Jenna Braddock for her knowledge of sports nutrition and her guidance on the foods that athletes need to be at their best, and my editors at Callisto Media, Anna Pulley and Michelle Anderson, who make my thoughts, ideas, and words shine.

Special praise goes to Eusebio Pareja and my team at Mexology and BKLYNwild, who keep my kitchens running smoothly so I can pursue writing projects.

Finally, as always, thanks to my family and friends, who are always there for love, support, and a laugh over a glass of wine. What would I do without you? And a special thank you to Diego and Frida, whose love and companionship I could never repay with any amount of dog treats.

About the Authors

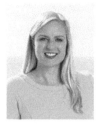

JENNA BRADDOCK is a registered dietitian nutritionist, certified specialist in sports dietetics, and ACSM certified personal trainer living in St. Augustine, Florida, with her husband, Brian, and two sons. Jenna's mission is to "Make Healthy Easy," so you have more space to live vibrantly and love others well. She specializes in behavior change counseling, performance nutrition, the Enneagram and eating, and enjoyable fitness. She has had the honor of working with individuals, groups, and companies to promote realistic, balanced health strategies, in addition to appearing regularly on TV and digital media outlets. In 2018, she launched OffSeasonAthlete.com, a website dedicated to providing teen athletes with safe and effective training information. To connect with Jenna, find her on Instagram at @Make.Healthy.Easy or JennaBraddock.com.

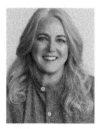

IVY STARK found her passion for food early on growing up in Boulder, Colorado, where she was first exposed to fine dining through her father, who worked in luxury hotel management. After earning her bachelor's degree in history at the University of California, Los Angeles, she attended Peter Kump's culinary school, now known as the Institute of Culinary Education, where she honed her culinary expertise in the professional studies program. Her first full-time position was at the award-winning Border Grill in Los Angeles, where she worked with Mary Sue Milliken and Susan Feniger.

Stark was the executive chef of the highly popular Mexican restaurant Dos Caminos in New York City, where she earned national recognition and ranked as one of New York's top chefs. During her time there, she oversaw all of the locations and played a pivotal role in the brand's expansion. It was there that she wrote her first book, *Dos Caminos Mexican Street Food: 120 Authentic Recipes to Make at Home*, which was published in 2013 and followed by *Dos Caminos Tacos* in 2014. She was nominated for the Women Chefs & Restaurateurs Golden Whisk Award.

In 2019, Ivy opened her own restaurants in Brooklyn: BKLYNwild, serving vegan and vegetarian food, and Mexology, serving fresh, creative Mexican food.

Printed in the USA
CPSIA information can be obtained
at www.ICGtesting.com
CBHW082019220524
8972CB00005B/70

9 781648 766688